MEDICAL DETECTIVES

MEDICAL DETECTIVES

The Lives & Cases of Britain's
FORENSIC FIVE

ROBIN ODELL

The
History
Press

Dedicated to the memory of Joe Gaute,
crime historian, publisher and friend.

First published 2013

The History Press
The Mill, Brimscombe Port
Stroud, Gloucestershire, GL5 2QG
www.thehistorypress.co.uk

British Library Cataloguing in Publication Data.
A catalogue record for this book is available from the British Library.

ISBN 978 0 7524 6449 7

Typesetting and origination by The History Press
Printed in India.

CONTENTS

Foreword by Professor Bernard Knight CBE   7

Acknowledgements   9

Introduction   10

About the Author   12

1 The Coming Man: Sir Bernard Spilsbury   13

2 The Patriarch: Sir Sydney Smith   62

3 The Professor: John Glaister   110

4 The Mentor: Francis Camps   144

5 The Teacher: Keith Simpson   171

Glossary   209

Bibliography   215

Index of Names   219

FOREWORD

by Professor Bernard Knight CBE

IN SPITE OF THE CURRENT OBSESSION of television producers portraying forensic pathologists as willowy blondes, aged twenty-five, this macabre occupation was dominated during the last century by a handful of mostly middle-aged or elderly men of all shapes and sizes, some of whom became 'household names'.

Robin Odell has taken five of the most prominent of these and expertly welded their personal histories to their most notorious cases, producing an engrossing record of how homicide was investigated during the twentieth century.

As it seemed almost obligatory for such men to write their memoirs – or have them 'ghosted' for them – much of the material has already been published, but some of these books have their faults. The early biography of Spilsbury. in 1951, was really an adulatory homage and it took until 2007 for Andrew Rose to write a more realistic assessment of the great man – and now Robin Odell has again offered a balanced view of Sir Bernard.

Though I knew of all five – and had met them all except Spilsbury during my half-century forensic career – my main interest was reading about Keith Simpson and Francis Camps, who I knew so well and whose personalities could not have been more different.

When I left the army to look for a job, I turned up at St Pancras mortuary one morning, still in uniform, and found Camps up to his elbows in a corpse, the inevitable fag in mouth, and was laconically told to 'start on Monday' with not even a mention of a salary! How different from the formal, immaculate Simpson, with his archbishop's voice that delivered superb lectures, compared with Camps' disjointed ramblings. Yet they both had their strengths and weaknesses, though their personal differences were sometimes too publicly ventilated.

Writing a biography of an eminent professional is not easy, as I found when I did that of Milton Helpern, the Chief Medical Examiner of New York City. It is hard to avoid trotting out a dry rehash of journalistic articles and court records, but Robin Odell, a veteran author of true crime, has imbued these pen-portraits with a true feeling of what the men were like, warts and all, offering a book that not only informs, but entertains.

ACKNOWLEDGEMENTS

I WISH TO THANK NON, as always, for her patience and encouragement. Grateful thanks are also extended to Andrew Rose for his support and advice, to Annie Hepburn who processed all the words, to David and Ann Tolley for checking them, and to Alan Greeley for his assistance with illustrations.

Every effort has been made to trace copyright holders of photographs but, in some instances, unsuccessfully. Where this is the case, acknowledgement is given to the original published source. I would also like to acknowledge the Joe Gaute archive of crime photographs and documents.

INTRODUCTION

THE DEVELOPMENT OF FORENSIC MEDICINE in Britain is told through the lives of the five great pathologists who dominated the scene throughout most of the twentieth century. Their careers spanned seventy years of personal achievement and innovation which laid the foundations of modern crime scene investigation.

Sir Bernard Spilsbury was an iconic figure who put forensic pathology on the map with his involvement in the Crippen case. Headlines such as, 'Spilsbury called in', turned an essentially shy man into a celebrity. He was in essence a loner; an interpreter who exemplified the role of the expert witness. Sure of himself, certain of the facts and not requiring a second opinion, he stood tall in the witness box. In an age when capital punishment was still in use, his courtroom testimony made him an arbiter of life and death. A roll call of his cases reads like a catalogue of famous British murders. His conclusions, though, were often controversial and contested and remain so to the present day. He was the epitome of the expert; aloof, assured and respected.

His contemporary, Sir Sydney Smith, by contrast, was an innovator, a clubbable man who worked on a broad canvas and drew people towards him. Born in New Zealand, he pursued his training in Scotland, the spiritual home of forensic medicine. He honed his skills in Egypt, where he worked during the inter-war years, and pioneered the development of forensic ballistics. He returned to Edinburgh to concentrate on teaching and helped to put forensic studies onto a sound academic basis.

John Glaister also prospered in the Scottish tradition and played a major role in furthering his nation's pre-eminent position in forensic medicine. He was a professor for thirty years at Glasgow University where he succeeded his father.

His particular contribution was to apply scientific methods to the examination of trace evidence gathered at crime scenes. His work on the identification of hair was a significant breakthrough and, like Smith, he was willing to share knowledge and to call for specialist help when it was needed. This was evident in the Ruxton case when he pioneered photo-imposition as an identification technique.

Francis Camps was an organiser rather than an innovator. He had a vision of coordinating the emerging skills of the broader medico-legal profession and, to that end, created a world-class forensic department at London University. He had his share of important crime cases but was at his best when managing people and resources to advance the knowledge and professional status of forensic work. He was a founding member of the British Academy of Forensic Sciences which succeeded in bringing science, medicine and the law together to serve the ends of justice. Camps also reached out to the USA to add an international element to what he viewed as best practice.

Keith Simpson combined a number of talents as teacher and practitioner. He was also an important innovator, breaking new ground in the understanding of factors which determined time of death and helping to put forensic dentistry on the map as a means of establishing identity. Like his contemporaries, he was involved in many headline murder cases, Heath, Haigh and Christie being prominent among them. He was a highly effective communicator, noted for his succinct delivery of evidence in court, in addition to his lecturing and writing activities.

The five pathologists, each with their unique talents, represented a golden age of forensic development. Their careers overlapped to a considerable extent and there were strains of rivalry in their relationships at times. This was, perhaps, inevitable in the adversarial system employed in British courts which meant that experts were sometimes cast as opponents in the courtroom. As professionals, they did not always agree on the interpretation of evidence.

Despite their differences, they elevated the gritty, not to say, gruesome, business of examining the dead to a multi-faceted profession calling on every available scientific resource and discipline. Crime scene investigation as it is practised today owes a great deal to these pioneers for their questing spirit and innovative genius.

Robin Odell, 2013

ABOUT THE AUTHOR

ROBIN ODELL has been writing books on true crime since the 1960s and is the author and co-author of twenty books covering criminal history and forensic investigation, and regularly lectures on the subject.

Chapter One

THE COMING MAN

Sir Bernard Spilsbury

THE THIRTY-THREE-YEAR-OLD MAN who stood in the witness box at the Old Bailey on 18 October 1910 was tall, good-looking and self-assured. He was well-dressed, sporting a red carnation in his buttonhole, and spoke clearly and calmly when addressed by counsel for the Crown. 'I am a Bachelor of Surgery of Oxford University and I hold the position of pathologist at St Mary's Hospital,' he told the court. The man was Bernard Spilsbury, whose name would become a household term epitomising the ascendancy of the medical detective, and the occasion was the trial for murder of Hawley Harvey Crippen whose name gained notoriety as a fashionable expletive.

Dr Spilsbury was the most junior of the four experts called by the prosecution to present the medical evidence against Crippen. His appearance was brief, decisive and memorable. From his high perch in the wood-panelled courtroom, the Lord Chief Justice, bewigged and swathed in scarlet, questioned the young pathologist about his opinion. Spilsbury, unintimidated, replied, 'I have an independent position of my own, and I am responsible for my own opinion, which has been formed on my own scientific knowledge . . . '. Those present who understood the workings of the medico-legal world realised at once that they were witnessing something important. A young law student at the time, who would later achieve fame as a coroner, Bentley Purchase, remembered people leaving the court and saying of Spilsbury, 'There is a coming man.'

Crippen was the inoffensive-looking husband of Kunigunde Mackamotski, a stage-struck woman better known as Cora or by her stage name, Belle Elmore.

The couple settled in England in 1900 after Crippen was appointed to run the London office of the Munyon Company, a Philadelphia-based patent medicine firm. Crippen's medical qualifications, described as obscure and probably acquired through the post, nevertheless allowed him to use the title of 'Dr'. It is doubtful, though, that he would have been allowed by the General Medical Council to practise in England. His success as a sales representative was matched by that of his wife as a stage artiste; he presided over dwindling fortunes selling quack medicine and she obtained minor parts in the music halls. Neighbours observed that he always appeared to be subservient to her wishes. Small in stature and mild in manner, his demeanour contrasted sharply with Cora's music-hall persona.

The Crippens lived at 39 Hilldrop Crescent in Camden Town in a gloomy house with a cellar. In January 1910, Crippen parted company with Munyons and began to run into debt. By this time, the little doctor was also running a double life with his teenage mistress, Ethel le Neve. They met secretly and shared warm embraces in the privacy of hotel bedrooms.

On 2 February 1910, Crippen told Ethel le Neve that his wife had gone to America. Ethel joined him at 39 Hilldrop Crescent and a couple of weeks later appeared at a charity ball wearing a brooch belonging to Cora Crippen. The doctor let it be known that he had heard his wife was seriously ill and he was planning to travel to the USA to be by her side. He then announced that she had died and, on the day that her obituary was published in the theatrical newspaper, *Era*, he and Ethel le Neve left England for a honeymoon in Dieppe. On 31 March, one of Cora's friends at the Music Hall Ladies' Group reported certain suspicions to Scotland Yard.

When Crippen and le Neve returned to Hilldrop Crescent it was to face visits from several of Cora's friends asking embarrassing questions and, finally, from Chief Inspector Walter Dew of Scotland Yard. This occurred at the beginning of July, weeks after Cora had disappeared. Crippen was disarmingly frank; 'The stories I have told about my wife's death are untrue,' he declared. He said that as far as he knew she was still alive and had gone to America to join her lover. He had lied, he explained, to hide his shame.

The policeman was thus put off the scent and Crippen, alerted to the danger he was in, prepared for flight. On 11 July, when Dew sought to question Crippen further, he found both the doctor's office and 39 Hilldrop Crescent unoccupied. The house was thoroughly searched and human remains were found buried in the cellar. The experts were called in and Dew took passage across the Atlantic in a ship fast enough to overhaul the SS *Montrose*, whose passengers included Crippen and le Neve dressed as a boy. An alert had been broadcast by wireless from the ship's captain to the owners in Liverpool. In an historic radio message, he said, 'Have strong suspicion that Crippen London Cellar Murderer and Accomplice are among saloon passengers ...'.

Under the brick floor of the cellar at the Crippen home, Dew and his Sergeant discovered the stinking remains of a human torso wrapped in a man's pyjama top. Augustus J. Pepper, consulting surgeon at St Mary's Hospital and a leading medico-legal authority, examined the cellar remains and reported that without question they were human. He called in his assistant, Dr Bernard Spilsbury, who sacrificed a holiday with his wife and son in Somerset for the doubtful privilege of evaluating the remains found at Hilldrop Crescent. Spilsbury's rising reputation had already been noted and it was said that Richard Muir, who prosecuted Crippen at his trial, especially asked for Spilsbury to work on the case.

The pathologist wrote out a summary of his initial findings on one of his famous record cards. Throughout his career he pursued the meticulous habit of recording the details of all his cases on record filing cards which at the end of his professional life numbered some 6,000. The discovery in the cellar amounted to a heap of putrefying flesh and organs; there was no head and no bones. When he was called to the scene, Sir Melville McNaghten, the Assistant Commissioner at Scotland Yard, had the foresight, as he recorded in his memoirs; 'to put a handful of cigars in my pocket; I thought they might be needed by the officers and they were!'

The sex of this grisly discovery was not apparent, for the genitalia were missing. All the organs of the chest and abdomen were accounted for with the exception of the reproductive organs. Later, on a section of skin measuring seven inches by six, which he thought came from the lower part of the abdomen, Pepper's experienced eye spotted a mark which he thought was a scar. This blemish was the cue for Spilsbury to step into the public arena.

The young Demonstrator of Pathology left his family to start their holiday without him while he remained in London and joined a forensic quartet at St Mary's Hospital – he and Pepper worked on the physical aspects of the remains while Dr William Willcox and Dr Arthur Luff carried out analyses for toxic substances. One of Spilsbury's three filing cards on Crippen recorded the essential information concerning the discovery in the cellar:

Human remains found July 13 . . . Medical organs of the chest and abdomen. Removed in one mass. Four large pieces of skin and muscle, one from the lower abdomen with old operation scar 4 in. long – broader at lower end. Impossible to identify sex. Hyoscine found 2.2 grains. Hair in Hinde's curler – roots present. Hair 6 in. long. Man's pyjama jacket, Jones Bros., Holloway, and odd pair of pyjama trousers.

Examined by Travers Humphreys, Spilsbury told the court how he had examined a piece of skin and flesh with a mark on it. 'I have formed the opinion,' he said, 'that it comes from the lower part of the wall of the abdomen, near the middle – I base that opinion upon the presence and arrangement of certain muscles.' Of the mark on the skin, he said, 'As the result of my microscopical examination I say that that mark is undoubtedly an old operation scar.' Knowing that Crippen's wife had undergone an ovarotomy in 1892 or '93, the identification of an abdominal surgical scar by the pathologist was an important plank in the prosecution's argument.

The thrust of Spilsbury's case was that the absence of hair follicles and sebaceous glands in the mark on the skin made it certain that it was a scar. He was at pains to point out that although he had been a student of Augustus Pepper, his opinions were entirely his own. He repeated, 'I think there is no room for doubt as to its being a scar,' and, as a final challenge, he declared, 'I have my microscope slides here and I shall send for a microscope in case it should be wanted.' Muir was no doubt very pleased with his protégé and took one of the defence's expert witnesses to task for daring to suggest that a mistake might have been made over interpretation of the microscopic evidence. 'We are not talking about people unaccustomed to the microscope,' declared counsel, 'we are talking about people like Mr Spilsbury.'

The sliver of tissue bearing the scar preserved in formalin in a glass dish was handed round among the members of the jury and, finally, in an adjoining room, Spilsbury set up his microscope so that any jurors who might have entertained lingering doubts could see his slides for themselves. The defence argument that the mark was merely a surface crease in the unbroken skin was weakened by the appearance of epithelium – the outermost layer of the skin – which had become folded into the scar as a result of the operation for ovarotomy.

Traces of hyoscine were found in the remains by Dr William Willcox; the presence of the drug linked to Crippen's known purchases of hyoscine hydrobromide from a chemist in New Oxford Street established cause of death and completed the chain of evidence. Willcox and Spilsbury were destined to work together on other important criminal cases; they made a formidable pair. The jury believed the remains found in the cellar at Hilldrop Crescent were those of Cora Crippen who had been poisoned by her husband. They took just half an hour to find him guilty of murder.

Spilsbury's precisely ordered mind was possibly a characteristic inherited from his father, an analytical and manufacturing chemist. James Spilsbury had wanted to train as a doctor but his mother was against the idea and urged him into a trade. The closest he could aspire to his real ambition was as a maker of pills and potions. James left his native Staffordshire in the 1870s and loosed the bonds of parental control. He set up in business in Leamington Spa where he married a local girl. In May 1877, James and Marion Spilsbury had the first of their four children, whom they named Bernard Henry.

Bernard was considered a handsome child, as photographs of the period testified, and he was cheerful and good-natured. The family home was comfortable and his father, who had suffered disappointment at not being allowed to follow the career of his own choosing, determined that, within reason, his children would be permitted to fulfil their particular talents and ambitions. Until he was ten years of age Bernard was tutored at home and, in 1888, enrolled as a pupil at Leamington College. He soon became a boarder for his father decided to shake the dust of the provinces from his feet and move to London. While James Spilsbury searched for a house in the metropolis that would be convenient for his new employment as consulting chemist to a number of large firms, he moved the rest of his family to his parents' home in Stafford.

A new family home was eventually found at Crouch End in north London and Bernard was reunited with his parents. But the move had no permanence, for Spilsbury senior's restlessness and quick business brain pinpointed an opportunity in Manchester and there the family moved at the end of 1891. Bernard attended Manchester Grammar School where, to his father's frustration, he performed only to a dull average but, with the benefits of hindsight, showed the languor and exasperating talent of a late developer. In 1893, he moved to Owens College where his career prospects began to come into focus.

He had decided he would like to train as a doctor and, two years later, took a step down that path when he passed his London University Matriculation. He subsequently gained entrance to Oxford University as a medical student.

His teachers at Owens College saw Bernard Spilsbury as something of a loner. He liked the solitude of long walks and preferred individual to team sports. The characteristic of the loner, tempered with a gritty determination, would stamp the young Spilsbury's future career.

The young man graduated with a BA degree from Oxford in 1899 after studying for three years at Magdalen College. With general practice in mind, he entered St Mary's Hospital Medical School at Paddington, London which would be a second home to him for twenty years. He at once came under the spell of two outstanding teachers, Arthur Luff and Augustus Pepper. He also fell in love with the microscope given to him by his father which became as indispensable to the large-as-life Spilsbury as the magnifying glass was to the mythical Sherlock Holmes.

Luff and Pepper have been described as the founders of modern forensic medicine but they had inherited a somewhat tarnished tradition owing to the fiasco created by the Smethurst trial in 1859. Dr Thomas Smethurst was charged with fatally poisoning Isabella Bankes, a spinster with whom he went to live after deserting his invalid wife. She left everything to Smethurst, whom she described as 'my sincere and beloved friend'.

Dr Alfred Swaine Taylor, the government analyst and a leading toxicologist, had found arsenic in the dead woman's body and also in a medicine bottle taken from the sickroom. On the basis of this evidence, Smethurst was sent for trial at the Old Bailey. Sensation occurred when Dr Taylor admitted that arsenical impurities in his test reagents invalidated his discovery of poison. Smethurst was nevertheless found guilty and was sentenced to be hanged. Because of the controversy over the toxicological analysis, the Home Office ordered an inquiry which resulted in Smethurst being pardoned and Taylor suffering the ignominy of an expert made fallible. In consequence, the standing of forensic medicine was severely dented and the *Dublin Medical Journal* wrote of poor Taylor that he had 'brought an amount of disrepute upon his branch of the profession that years will not remove'.

Following this debacle, the role of the expert witness was held in some suspicion and it fell to St Mary's Hospital to reinstate what some called a 'beastly science' to its rightful place. Spilsbury's tutors encouraged their student's enthusiasm for microscopy, perhaps seeing his potential for enhancing their calling. Spilsbury's natural aloofness and liking for solitary working predisposed him to the pursuit of pathology. At any rate, he chose that calling and, as his contemporaries all observed, devoted himself diligently to his studies. This decision had the effect of concentrating the young man's individualistic tendencies and he was drawn to the professional company of older men. His fellow students doubtless thought he had a high opinion of himself.

The late developer found that some of those medical students who had started their studies after him qualified before he did. But in 1905, at the age of twenty-eight, he graduated from Oxford with his medical degree. In the same year, he became engaged to Edith Horton whom he had met in Birmingham four years earlier while visiting his itinerant parents. In October 1905, Dr Bernard Spilsbury was appointed Resident Assistant Pathologist at St Mary's under Augustus Pepper. His appointment completed a formidable team; Pepper was the Home Office pathologist and Arthur Luff was joint toxicologist to the Home Office with William Willcox, a man only a few years older than Spilsbury and a natural ally. They were to become good friends and worked together professionally on many important cases.

Spilsbury, now earning a salary of £200 a year, was thus put into the arena where the reputation of modern forensic pathology would be moulded. He had access not only to the best knowledge and experience available but also to those meticulous working disciplines so vital in the medico-legal world. Within six years, he would come to the forefront of the national scene, his name a public property, while many of those who outshone him as students remained in respectable obscurity.

He was able to augment his salary with earnings from coroners' fees which, in those days, ran to two guineas for a post-mortem examination. His first fee-earning post-mortem was performed in March 1906. It rated an entry on one of his famous record cards which, together with his notebooks, were maintained as material for an eventual text-book on forensic medicine.

Spilsbury lived at rooms in Cambridge Terrace, Paddington, not quite 'over the shop' but within easy reach of St Mary's. By 1908, the demand for his services outside the hospital was so great that he was serving several coroners' courts in London and earning fees which doubled his salary. He managed his income carefully, having decided to marry Edith Horton when he had settled into his professional career. He judged that moment to have arrived in 1908 and in September the couple were married at Moseley. They rented a house at Harrow-on-the-Hill in north London and Spilsbury commuted to Paddington each day on the newly electrified Metropolitan Railway. The following year, he succeeded Augustus Pepper as Pathologist at St Mary's when his friend and tutor retired. His rise had been fast by any standard and then came the Crippen trial.

The Crippen case was a watershed for Spilsbury. It was a signpost on a road to a unique career which embraced a dozen at least of the most sensational murder cases in the history of English crime. His appearance at the Old Bailey to give expert testimony fixed his name and personality in the minds of the public at a time when reports of the great criminal trials attracted massive newspaper readership. It was a time before charisma had been invented but there was no doubt that Spilsbury had that indefinable quality which would mark him out as a figure commanding public attention.

As with many charismatic figures, providence provided Spilsbury with material for the proper exercise of his talent. In the wake of the Crippen trial, Augustus Pepper decided to withdraw from public life and recommended Spilsbury to succeed him as Home Office pathologist. This meant working as assistant to Willcox who was now Senior Home Office pathologist. Willcox welcomed the new appointment and so began an outstanding professional partnership that lasted for nearly thirty years. By a strange paradox, the last engagements of the two men included courtroom appearances on opposing sides. But what lay before them in 1911 was a succession of extraordinary criminal cases which began in September of that year with another murder in north London.

Frederick Henry Seddon lived with his wife and their five children at 63 Tollington Park, Islington less than a mile away from the former residence of the Crippens. Seddon was a district superintendent for the London and Manchester Industrial Assurance Company. After he was promoted in 1909, he moved his family into a better district, taking a lease on a three-storey house. He used the basement front room as an office and the safe which he installed there frequently contained large sums of money which he took in from the collectors whom he supervised. Seddon charged the insurance company 5s a week for the use of part of his house as an office. A fascination for money was his singular characteristic; he loved the chore of counting the gold and silver into little piles on his desk. It was said of him that gold was his god and that his temple was the Finsbury Park branch of the London and Provincial Bank.

An unhealthy love of money for its own sake not unnaturally inspired greed and meanness. He charged his teenage sons for their board and lodgings and he decided to put the spare accommodation at his house to good use by advertising for a lodger. The successful applicant was Eliza Mary Barrow, a forty-nine-year-old spinster, who took the upper rooms for 12s 6d a week. Seddon's tenant was a somewhat eccentric person who moved in with a retinue of three retainers to look after her needs. With his talent for meanness, Seddon immediately recognised a similar trait in Eliza Barrow. She too liked the miser's feel of money and kept considerable sums of gold in a box in her room. He also discovered that she had interests in property and owned large investments.

Two of Miss Barrow's companions left after an argument with Seddon and only Ernie Grant, a ten-year-old orphan, remained to do her bidding. Seddon now stepped into a protective role, offering the services of his sixteen-year-old daughter at a shilling a day to look after her. He also offered to put her cashbox in his basement safe in order to provide better security for her savings which he soon ascertained amounted to £400 in gold and bank notes.

By an insidious process of persistent questioning and probing, Seddon obtained a complete evaluation of Miss Barrow's income from property and investments. Little by little, he persuaded her, over a period of fourteen months, to transfer all her assets to his management. The arrangement was that in return for assuming the burden and responsibility of maintaining her affairs, he would grant her a life annuity of £52. All was harmony it seemed and in the summer of 1911, the Seddons took Eliza Barrow with them on holiday to Southend.

On their return to Tollington Park, life returned to normal except that in an exceptionally hot summer the Seddon household was troubled with flies. Mrs Seddon bought a supply of arsenical fly-papers from the nearby chemist shop at the bargain price of four for three pence. At the time, Miss Barrow was suffering a bilious attack and she was bothered by flies in her bedroom. Mrs Seddon very kindly put the fly-papers in saucers and added some water in the prescribed manner. She placed two on the mantelshelf and two on the chest of drawers.

Miss Barrow's bilious attack was of long duration and by 5 September necessitated daily visits by the doctor, who was concerned at the weakness caused in his patient by continuous sickness and diarrhoea. By 12 September there was further deterioration and the doctor became anxious, indicating that he thought Miss Barrow was in some danger. Mrs Seddon stayed the night with her and fell asleep in the chair. When she awoke, she found Miss Barrow lying stiff in bed – she had died in the early hours of the morning. The doctor was informed and he issued a death certificate without seeing the body. Cause of death was given as 'epidemic diarrhoea'.

Frederick Seddon's first action was to search for the keys to the trunk which contained all the dead woman's worldly goods – at least those which he had not already wheedled out of her. With his eagle eye for hidden treasure, he next searched the room and turned up a few sovereigns here and a few coppers there. His second action was to visit the undertaker and beat him down on price to £3 7s 6d for what the funeral parlour described as a 'nice turnout'. True to form, Seddon took 12s 6d as his commission on the deal. Eliza Barrow went to her grave with few mourners. Ironically, she was buried at Islington Borough Cemetery at Finchley where, less than twelve months previously, Cora Crippen's remains had been laid to rest. It proved to be no last resting place for Eliza Barrow, for within a few weeks her body was exhumed for examination by Doctors Spilsbury and Willcox.

Suspicion was first aroused by the dead woman's cousin, Frank Vonderhahe, who called at the Seddons' home. After a somewhat strained interview in which Seddon refused to impart any information regarding the late Eliza Barrow's financial affairs or to produce her will, Vonderhahe voiced certain nagging doubts to the authorities. The Director of Public Prosecutions decided that further investigation was required and granted an exhumation order. Miss Barrow's body was disinterred on 15 November and Spilsbury carried out a post-mortem examination. His record card noted that the internal organs were 'extremely well-preserved' and that 'no disease was apparent'. The remarkable state of preservation after nine weeks of burial was characteristic of arsenical poisoning.

Establishing the exact cause of death fell to Willcox, aided by John Webster, the Home Office analyst. Mindful of the furore created by Taylor in 1859, the analysts had been working on a modified method of analysing for arsenic which was both quick and accurate. Their qualitative test, used for the first time in the Seddon case, became the standard procedure and was used as such for nearly thirty years. The amount of arsenic found in the organs of Miss Barrow's body was estimated at 131.57 milligrams (2.01 grains) and the total content in the body would have amounted to considerably more. The presence of arsenic in the hair and fingernails indicated that the poison had been ingested during a period of about two weeks prior to death. In light of this information, the coroner's inquest reached a verdict of 'death due to arsenical poisoning administered by some person or persons unknown'. A warrant was issued for the arrest of Frederick Seddon and he was apprehended in the street near his home on 4 December.

Frederick and Margaret Seddon were tried at the Old Bailey in March 1912, the proceedings being noted for the presence of a number of illustrious legal figures. In keeping with tradition in cases of poisoning, the prosecution was led by the Attorney-General, Sir Rufus Isaacs, a future Lord Chief Justice of England. He was assisted by two other counsel who would reach great distinction, Richard Muir and Travers Humphreys. The defence was headed by Edward Marshall Hall and Mr Justice Bucknill presided over what, for the time, was a long trial lasting ten days. The trial was unusual too in that both defendants, man and wife, faced a capital charge involving one set of evidence, most of which was circumstantial.

Spilsbury, elegant in both dress and manner, was first into the witness box for the Crown. Under examination by the Attorney-General he related his chief post-mortem finding which was the remarkable state of preservation of the body. He described the condition as 'very abnormal' and added, 'I was not able to account for it at the time the post-mortem examination was made, but since the analysis which has been made by Dr Willcox I think the preservation was due to the presence of arsenic in the body.'

Apart from some reddening of the intestines, he had found no sign whatever of any disease. He agreed that death might have resulted from syncope or heart failure. The inflammation of the intestine, considered in the absence of disease in any other organ, would, he agreed, be equally indicative of death due to epidemic diarrhoea. But, there was the evidence of the unusual preservation of the body to be taken into account. All things considered, he believed the post-mortem evidence was more consistent with acute arsenical poisoning than with any other cause of death that had been suggested.

Seeking an alternative explanation for the state of preservation, defence counsel brought up the time-honoured phenomenon of the arsenic-eating peasants of the Styria region in Hungary. The Styrian habit of regularly eating arsenic and thereby acquiring immunity to its toxic effects was invariably raised at trials for poisoning by arsenic. It was introduced at Seddon's trial by the defence in an attempt to show that Eliza Barrow died not from acute poisoning as argued by Spilsbury but from chronic poisoning. The implication was that Miss Barrow had been ingesting arsenic over a long period perhaps to improve her complexion by acquiring a pink glow to her skin in the manner suggested by Florence Maybrick to be the fashion in the 1880s. Consequently, it was suggested that, while she had arsenic in her body, and her corpse was well-preserved, she did not die of arsenical poisoning.

Spilsbury said that the body showed no features indicating that arsenic had been given over a prolonged period. He agreed with Willcox that about 5 grains had been ingested within three days of death and that a similar amount had probably preceded it. Attempts by the defence to move Spilsbury away from the acute poisoning explanation of Miss Barrow's death failed completely. When Willcox went into the witness box, Marshall Hall asked him, '. . . taking the result of your various analyses, tests and examinations, what do you say was the cause of Miss Barrow's death?' Back came the unequivocal reply, 'Acute arsenical poisoning.'

As part of his preparation for the case, Willcox carried out various tests with Mather's fly-papers of the type found in the Seddons' house. Each paper contained between 3.8 and 6.0 grains of arsenic – well in excess of the fatal dose of 2.0 grains. The arsenic could be leached out of the papers by pouring boiling water over them and leaving them to soak overnight. It was known that Miss Barrow had frequently drunk brandy as a medicinal aid during her illness. The spirit would have been an ideal medium in which to dispense a dose of tasteless and odourless solution of arsenic.

Marshall Hall rightly pointed out that there was not a shred of evidence that either of the Seddons had ever boiled a fly-paper. But the overall power of the circumstantial evidence was heightened by Frederick Seddon's portrayal of greed and, hence, of motive, when he answered the Attorney-General's questions. In his final speech for the Crown, Sir Rufus Isaacs appealed to the court's idealism by referring not only to the content but also the tone of the testimony given by Spilsbury and Willcox. There was something about the way Spilsbury projected himself which inspired admiring references to his honesty. If he was embarrassed by such comment he did not show it sufficiently to prevent its repetition throughout his career.

As the Seddon trial drew to a close, Sir Rufus Isaacs said, 'I would like in passing to say this, that in the course of a very long experience at the Bar I never remember hearing witnesses give evidence as Dr Willcox and Dr Spilsbury did, with more impartiality and more honesty in every word they uttered.' This fulsome praise from the man who in less than a year would be appointed Lord Chief Justice of England, represented not only a great compliment to the two men concerned but it also marked a renaissance of forensic medicine.

In his closing speech, Sir Edward Marshall Hall argued for a reconstruction of events at 63 Tollington Park that allowed the possibility of Miss Barrow accidentally administering the fatal arsenic to herself. Counsel constructed an ingenious if unconvincing account of the way in which this might have occurred. But it was all too late. Seddon had already left an indelible impression on the jury and junior counsel, Gervais Rentoul, commented that when he went into the witness box 'one felt that the shadow of the gallows had crept appreciably nearer'. The jury found Frederick Seddon guilty and his wife, Margaret, not guilty. The final drama came when Seddon was asked the traditional question, 'Have you anything to say for yourself why the court should not give you the judgement of death according to law?'

'I have, sir,' came the answer, and Seddon treated the court to an extraordinary address in which he reviewed and repudiated the evidence brought against him.

In a poignant conclusion to a remarkable trial, Seddon, a Freemason, declared his innocence before the Great Architect of the Universe. This so moved Mr Justice Bucknill, himself a member of the Brotherhood, that he had difficulty controlling his emotions. With tears wetting his face, he pronounced sentence of death and advised Seddon to try to make peace with his Maker. 'I am at peace,' retorted the condemned man, as the judge fumbled his way through to the end of the prescribed litany.

Marshall Hall described Frederick Seddon as 'The ablest man I ever defended on a capital charge'. Spilsbury, in his copy of *The Trial of the Seddons* in the Notable British Trials series, marked passages in the text of Marshall Hall's speeches which criticised the prosecution's evidence, especially its circumstantial nature.

After the consecutive sensations of the Crippen and Seddon trials, Spilsbury was able to settle down to a quieter routine, although his workload had increased as rapidly as his fame. While he started to consolidate his already successful career, another man destined for greatness in the world of forensic medicine had just qualified at Edinburgh. Sydney Smith, an eventual Professor of Forensic Medicine at Edinburgh University, but in 1912 a newly qualified doctor unsure of his future, followed the forensic trail more by accident than career choice. Like Spilsbury, he was talent-spotted by one of the great pioneers, Professor Harvey Littlejohn, then Dean of the Faculty of Medicine at Edinburgh.

In the course of their separate and distinguished careers, Spilsbury and Smith would confront each other as opposing experts in a criminal trial, but that was still a long way off. Edith Spilsbury was expecting their second child and her husband had aspirations of creating his own laboratory. With these factors in mind, the Spilsburys moved in 1912 to a larger house. They took up residence in a large semi-detached house in St John's Wood.

It proved to be a worrying time, for Edith required an emergency operation for appendicitis a few weeks before her baby was due. The surgery was successful, as was the childbirth, but her infant son, Alan, was a child of delicate health. When family life returned to normal, Spilsbury was able to devote some of his time to his pet project in one of the spare bedrooms of his new home. There he began to establish a laboratory so that he could continue working in his own time while keeping close to his family.

Of course, a forensic pathologist's career is not composed entirely of sensational murder cases which create large newspaper headlines and end with a criminal trial. There were in Spilsbury's time, as there are now, numerous deaths occasioned by accident, suicide or murder for which there is no immediately apparent explanation. It is the job of the forensic pathologist, acting as a kind of medical detective, to find an adequate cause of death. In performing this role, he satisfies not only the sophisticated medico-legal code established by civilised societies but also the instinctive need which the human race recognises for every death of one of its members to be properly explained.

In the course of his career and chiefly through the medium of the post-mortem examination, Spilsbury became acquainted with death in a myriad of forms. They varied from the bizarre to the simply tragic and, with each, came an explanation to satisfy the law and a contribution to his knowledge and experience. Spilsbury kept detailed notes of his work and also maintained a separate filing card system on which he recorded individual cases. His intention was, ultimately, to distil the carefully recorded information of a professional career into a text-book. Sadly, he never achieved this, so that the world was deprived of the insight which the man's own words on the printed page would have conveyed.

The vagaries of crime and the complexities of the human body combined to provide Spilsbury with fascinating fields of enquiry. In January 1914, he examined the body of five-year-old Willie Starchfield who had been found murdered in a railway carriage at Broad Farm. The contents of the boy's stomach provided useful evidence in this case by corroborating a witness's sighting of him eating a piece of cake on the day he was murdered. Analysis of stomach contents and an evaluation of the rate of digestion are used in modern forensic investigation to help determine the time of death.

Spilsbury was also interested in *contre coup* injuries and their possible relevance to brain tumours. *Contre coup* damage to the brain occurs on the side opposite to the point of a violent impact when the brain bounces against the inside of the skull. He believed that non-fatal injuries of this kind might subsequently trigger the growth of a tumour. When he had the opportunity, he took brain sections at his autopsies which were destined for microscopic examination in his laboratory.

When the Great War erupted, Spilsbury's offer to serve was turned down by the War Office. While his friend, William Willcox, disintinguished himself in the Royal Army Medical Corps, reorganising the Indian Medical Service in Mesopotamia, Spilsbury remained at the home front. He was by this time an essential part of the medico-legal establishment and it was felt that his work was indispensable. The penalty for those professional men and women not called for military service was to take on a greater burden to compensate for those who were absent. Not that Spilsbury escaped the war entirely, for some of those killed in Germany's Zeppelin raids on London in 1915 featured in his case records.

While his fellow countrymen were fighting and dying in the trenches in France, one George Joseph Smith was busy with those pursuits which would earn him the name of 'The Brides in the Bath Murderer'. Smith, who shared something of Seddon's love of money and also a streak of meanness, began his bigamous depradations in 1910. By January 1915, he had married three times and lost each bride through a tragic bathroom drowning. On each occasion, Smith's grief was partially ameliorated by the acquisition of his late bride's worldly wealth.

On Sunday, 3 January 1915, the *News of the World* published a story with the headline, 'FOUND DEAD IN BATH', which was an account of a young woman's accidental death by drowning. Among the millions who read the newspaper report was Charles Burnham who lived at Aston Clinton in Buckinghamshire and Joseph Crossley, whose mother let rooms in Blackpool.

Both men reacted sharply and reached for pen and paper to write to the authorities advising them of certain facts. Burnham's daughter, Alice, had drowned in the bath at Mrs Crossley's boarding house in Blackpool in December 1913. Her husband, George Joseph Smith, was mentioned in the newspaper report as being married to Margaret Lofty who met a 'tragic fate on the day after her wedding'. The local police forces, alerted by Burnham and Crossley, conferred with Scotland Yard, and Detective Inspector Arthur Fowler Neil was assigned to the investigation. Nationwide enquiries were made which resulted in suspicion being levelled at Smith in respect of three accidental drownings; Bessie Mundy at Herne Bay in July 1910, Alice Burnham at Blackpool in November 1913 and Margaret Lofty in London in December 1914.

Smith was arrested on 4 February 1915, on the same day that Spilsbury attended the cemetery at Finchley to oversee the exhumation of Margaret Lofty's body. Finchley Cemetery was beginning to feature regularly in his records – the remains of both Crippen's and Seddon's victims reposed there. Within the next fortnight he carried out similar missions at Blackpool and Herne Bay. On 23 March, Smith was charged with committing three murders, already dubbed by the press as 'The Brides in the Bath' case. Despite the war news from France, the newspapers found ample space to devote to the activities of Mr Smith. Come the trial, he was required to answer one murder charge only, that relating to Bessie Mundy at Herne Bay.

Smith met Beatrice Constance Annie Mundy, the thirty-three-year-old daughter of a bank manager, in Bristol. At the time, he presented himself as a picture restorer and immediately won over the rather shy Miss Mundy. In fact, Smith had only recently left his wife, Edith, at Southend where they had bought a house. When he met Bessie Mundy, he was searching out possible new sources of funding and who better than the daughter of a recently deceased bank manager who received £8 a month from a trust fund? On 26 October 1910, the couple were married at Weymouth Registry Office. Within a few weeks, having gained access to Bessie's money, Smith took his leave. He wrote her a cruel letter accusing her of blighting his future by giving him a disease which he called 'the bad disorder'.

Eighteen months later and quite by chance, Smith encountered Bessie on the seafront at Weston-super-Mare. Overcome with joy, she took him back to the boarding house where she was staying and announced that she had found her husband. Despite the cruel accusations made in his letters, reconciliation followed and the couple left Weston-super-Mare living as itinerants for three months before settling at Herne Bay in Kent. They rented a small house in the High Street and Smith put up a brass plate announcing that 'H.W. Williams, Art Dealer', was in business in the town.

Smith's movements were carefully planned. On 8 July 1912, he visited a solicitor and had wills drawn up for Mr and Mrs H. Williams. The effect of this was that in the event of the death of one of the parties, the other would inherit the assets of the deceased. This seemed a sensible arrangement except for the fact that, while Smith possessed little of value, Bessie was worth £2,500. The day after the wills were drawn up, Smith went on a shopping expedition – his object was to purchase a bath. This appeared to be another sensible move, for their accommodation lacked the amenity of a bathroom and Bessie had expressed the wish that they should buy one. Smith and Bessie found an ironmonger offering for sale a second-hand bath priced at £2. Bessie liked it and persuaded the shopkeeper to let it go for £1 17s 6d, doubtless much to the amusement and delight of her husband. The bath was delivered and installed on the same day.

On 10 July, 'Mr and Mrs Williams' asked for an appointment with one of the town's medical practitioners. Dr Frank French was told that Bessie had suffered a fit the previous day during which she lost consciousness. The doctor examined her but found nothing obviously wrong. He prescribed a mild sedative. Two days later, 'Williams' requested Dr French to visit his wife at home where she was in bed following another attack. Again the doctor's examination produced no startling results and he promised to call again later in the day. When he paid his second visit, he received no reply and was about to leave when 'Mr and Mrs Williams' appeared in the street. As Dr French reported later, 'Mrs Williams seemed to be in perfect health,' but the following morning he was sent a note by 'Williams' which read, 'Can you come at once? I am afraid my wife is dead.'

When he called at the house, Dr French was ushered into one of the upstairs rooms by 'Williams'. In the centre of the room stood a bath, three parts full of water in which Bessie lay, face upwards; there was no discernible pulse. With assistance from 'Williams' the doctor lifted the woman out of the bath and onto the floor where he attempted artificial respiration. His efforts at revival failed and he pronounced Bessie dead. The only witness at the coroner's inquest was 'Williams', who sobbed throughout the proceedings, and Dr French. The coroner remarked that he could see no evidence on which to censure 'Williams' and a verdict was returned of death by misadventure. The conclusion was that Bessie had suffered an epileptic seizure while taking a bath and as a result she fell back into the water and drowned. Her grieving husband made the necessary funeral arrangements and, before taking his leave of Herne Bay, persuaded the ironmonger who had sold him the bath to take it back. The shopkeeper obligingly met this request not least because he had received no payment in the first place. Probate was granted on the late 'Mrs Williams's' will in September 1912 and Smith, richer by £2,500, re-joined his real wife. He explained that he had been on a visit to Canada where he had made money dealing in porcelain.

Thanks to two astute newspaper readers, Smith's game plan was rumbled but not before he had drowned two more brides in their baths. When he exhumed Bessie Mundy's body on 19 February 1915, Bernard Spilsbury reported, 'I am of the opinion that we have not, so far, discovered the full list of this man's crimes.' When Smith was eventually arraigned before the magistrates at Bow Street, he was committed on three charges of murder and, in due course, was tried in respect of the death of Bessie Mundy.

While the newspapers were filled with news of the Dardanelles campaign, Smith had helped to ensure continued public interest by his outburst at Bow Street when he accused the Crown counsel, Archibald Bodkin, of being a criminal and a 'manufacturer of criminals'. The public sensed that the trial of this man would be no ordinary affair and they were right, for the murder trial of George Joseph Smith proved to be the longest in England since that of the notorious poisoner, William Palmer, in 1856.

Smith was defended at the Old Bailey by Edward Marshall Hall and the prosecution was in the hands of Archibald Bodkin whose expert witnesses were Doctors Spilsbury and Willcox. All four men were rising to the peak of their powers and stood on the edge of great achievements. For Willcox, shortly to be posted on military duties in the Dardanelles, this was his last important trial as Home Office pathologist. He had been called by the Home Secretary to see whether drugs had played any part in what otherwise appeared to be three cases of drowning. His analyses uncovered no traces of drugs or poison in the exhumed bodies and the way was thus opened up for Spilsbury to appear on centre stage as the Crown's principal expert witness.

Marshall Hall failed in his attempt to have the evidence of the other deaths ruled inadmissible when Smith was only charged with a single murder. Archibald Bodkin, in a brilliant piece of advocacy, laid out the case against Smith and by carefully listing the points of similarity between the three drownings, demonstrated that more than simple coincidence had been at work. Spilsbury's entrance was preceded by the appearance in the courtroom of two baths as exhibits. Not surprisingly, this event created a stir when the instruments of death were placed close to the solicitors' table.

Bodkin questioned Spilsbury and took him through his post-mortem findings on the three exhumed bodies. He had found no trace of disease in Bessie Mundy nor in Margaret Lofty; in the case of Alice Burnham, there was a slight thickening of one of the heart valves, although not serious enough to endanger her life. Turning to the two baths in whose shallow depths Bessie and Alice had died, Spilsbury proceeded in his precise and confident style to explain.

Firstly, he disposed of the epilepsy theory of Bessie Mundy's demise. 'In view of her height, five feet seven inches, and the length of the bath, five feet, I do not think her head would be submerged,' he said of the early stage of an epileptic fit when the body tends to become rigid. 'The head end of this bath is sloping,' he continued, 'and if her feet were against the narrow end when the body was rigid, it would tend to thrust the head up and out of the bath.' In the second stage of a fit, when the body contracts, Spilsbury thought that the lower part of the trunk would be resting on the bottom of the bath and therefore it was unlikely that the body would move down to the foot end of the bath sufficiently to submerge the head. After the seizure had run its course, the body would be limp and unconscious. 'I do not think,' he said, 'that she would be likely to be immersed during the stage of relaxation, because the sloping part at the head and bottom of the bath would support the upper part of the trunk and head.'

Referring to Dr French's report of finding the dead woman in the bath with her legs stretched out straight and the feet out of the water, Spilsbury said, 'I cannot give any explanation of how a woman – assuming she has had an epileptic seizure – could get into that position by herself.' He added, 'If the feet at the narrow end were lifted out of the water that might allow the trunk and head to slide down the bath.'

Spilsbury had considered all the possible scenarios for accidental drowning in the bath. Indeed these had all been discussed with Willcox beforehand and the two men were in complete agreement. The consequences of a person sitting in a bath and fainting would result in the body becoming limp and falling backwards. He believed that if water was thereby taken in through the mouth or nose, the effect would be to stimulate a return to consciousness. He admitted that a person kneeling or standing while taking a bath might pitch forward and, in consequence, be drowned. But as he pointed out, 'the body would be lying face downwards in the water.' In short, having taken accurate measurements of the three baths and considered the height of the three victims of drowning, the irrevocable conclusion was that their deaths were assisted by human intervention. The small size of the baths effectively ruled out the possibility of accidental drowning.

Following one of their pre-trial meetings, Spilsbury and Willcox considered the likely course of events on the brides' fateful bath nights. Willcox's notes summarised their views:

Q. Was drowning accidental? e.g. fit or syncope, followed by asphyxia?

A. From evidence we think 'No'.

Q. Was death suicide?

A. No evidence of suicidal tendencies in these cases, nor of mental instability.

Q. Was death homicidal?

A. We think, 'Right hand on head of woman, left forearm of assailant beneath both knees, left forearm of assailant suddenly raised while right hand is pressed down on head of woman. Then the trunk of body slides down towards the foot end of the bath, the head being submerged in water.'

During a break in court proceedings, Inspector Neil carried out an experiment in the presence of the jury to demonstrate the theory with the cooperation of a nurse dressed in a bathing costume. He applied the method postulated by Spilsbury and Willcox with startling results, for the volunteer had to be revived by means of artifical respiration. Spilsbury's biographers recorded his disapproval of the experiment, but if there were any lingering doubts as to the method most likely to have been employed by Smith to despatch his brides, this demonstration must have dispelled them.

As he had done at Bow Street Magistrates' Court, Smith made several interventions. When his defence advisers attempted to calm him, he turned on them too, but he saved most of his heckling for Mr Justice Scrutton's summing-up. 'You may as well hang me at once, the way you're going on,' he shouted. 'It's a disgrace to a Christian country, this is. I am not a murderer, though I may be a bit peculiar.' The summing-up consumed nearly a whole day in court and the judge gave instructions that the infamous baths should be placed in a basement room of the court building so that the jury could take another look at them. The jury was out for a mere twenty minutes before returning to announce a guilty verdict.

Smith's appeal was turned down and he was executed at Maidstone on 13 August 1915. Stuart Wood, in his memoirs *Shades of the Prison House*, gave an account of Smith's passage to the gallows. Wood was an inmate at Maidstone at the time and pressed his ear to his cell door as Smith was taken to the execution shed. He heard the sound of laboured breathing, of men supporting a heavy burden, and concluded that Smith was in a state of collapse.

Marshall Hall had been uncharacteristically subdued during the trial. He was up against a masterly presentation of evidence by Bodkin and, having failed to shift Spilsbury on any point of his testimony, must have known he faced a lost cause. His final speech was impressive, though, and he made much of the lack of marks of violence on the victims, arguing that their absence showed lack of proof against the accused man. But in all truth, Spilsbury's careful reconstruction had shown how easy it was for an unsuspecting victim in a bath tub to be placed at a helpless disadvantage by a scheming murderer. Once the legs had been pulled up and the head drawn down beneath the water there was little the victim could do but thresh about until asphyxiation ensued. With an operator of the calibre of Smith, the only indications of a struggle were likely to be water splashes on the floor.

After the trial of George Joseph Smith, Willcox went off to Mesopotamia and Spilsbury remained at home discharging an ever-growing number of cases. His family moved to Malvern at the time of the Zeppelin raids on London which allowed him to work a fierce regime, often including Sundays. With laboratory facilities at Marlborough Hill, he was able to work on post-mortem specimens at home and he burned the midnight oil more than was wise. His relaxation came through walking and the occasional game of tennis. It was not a healthy lifestyle and in 1917 he contracted an infection in his left arm after carrying out a post-mortem on a badly decomposed corpse. He was ordered to rest but like many medical men, he found it difficult to obey doctor's orders. By now, his family had grown and Edith had three children under the age of seven to look after.

There was no let-up in Spilsbury's workload during the war years and the pathologist had the unusual experience in the Voisin case of giving evidence to a jury using mime. Louis Voisin, a French butcher living in London, murdered his mistress, Emilienne Gerard, and, having dismembered her body, distributed the parcelled-up pieces around Bloomsbury. Voisin and another lady friend, Berthe Roche, were charged with murder and tried at the Old Bailey in 1918. He was convicted and sentenced to death and she was remanded to be charged as an accessory after the fact.

According to Spilsbury's reconstruction of the crime, it was clear that Roche had led the violence which resulted in Mme Gerard's death. The attack had taken place in the basement of 101 Charlotte Street where the blood patterns on walls and floor spoke eloquently enough to the pathologist. But when Mr Justice Avory instructed the jury to visit the room, Spilsbury was told to remain silent in order not to prejudice the trial. Accordingly, he went through a mime, graphically demonstrating how the murder had been committed and pointing out the distribution of blood spatters. The jury found Voisin guilty and he was hanged, while Berthe Roche was found guilty as an accessory and was sentenced to seven years' imprisonment. She did not see out her sentence, though, due to her death in a hospice in May 1919.

Spilsbury's reputation was made well before the end of the Great War in 1918. His involvement in important murder trials and emergence as a public figure no doubt created professional jealousy among some of his colleagues. The confidence which was characteristic of the man had been strengthened by his success. The coming man had certainly arrived and, in some quarters, his confidence was probably mistaken for arrogance and Spilsbury's preference for keeping his own counsel provoked some resentment.

As frequently happens, smouldering ill-feeling erupted from a trivial cause. In 1919, a member of the medical staff at St Mary's asked Spilsbury to preserve a specimen for him. In his view the item in question did not merit preserving and he offered that opinion. His assessment was not well received and his colleague told him that he should do as he was asked. Not surprisingly, Spilsbury reacted unfavourably to such cavalier treatment and demanded an apology. Thus, a small incident was blown up out of all proportion and when no apology was forthcoming, the matter was referred to the hospital's Court of Governors, which set up an enquiry.

Before any decision was reached, Spilsbury tendered his resignation and, on 18 November 1919, broke his twenty-year long association with St Mary's. His great friend, William Willcox, was embarrassed by the affair but felt that no good would be achieved by attempting to intervene. In the event, the court of enquiry found in Spilsbury's favour and the other participant in the incident was instructed to apologise.

The 1920s opened with Spilsbury starting a new appointment as Lecturer on Morbid Anatomy and Histology at St Bartholomew's Hospital and he carried on his work virtually without interruption. The break with St Mary's must have been a sad moment for him, but, happily, it did not affect his friendships, especially that which he enjoyed with Willcox. The two men shared the habit of working late at night and frequently met either at Willcox's home or in Spilsbury's laboratory at Marlborough Hill to discuss current cases.

The decade began with two remarkable poisoning cases which shared a number of common features. Both occurred in Wales, both involved arsenical poisoning and in both cases the individual accused was a practising solicitor. The first resulted in the acquittal of Harold Greenwood at Carmarthen in 1920 when he was brilliantly defended by Sir Edward Marshall Hall; the second ended in the conviction of Major Herbert Rowse Armstrong at Hereford in 1922. Willcox was consulted in both cases, while Spilsbury was involved only in the investigation of Major Armstrong's crime.

Armstrong was arrested on 31 December 1921 at his office in Hay-on-Wye following a high-level meeting between Sir William Willcox, who had been knighted earlier in the year, and Sir Archibald Bodkin, the Director of Public Prosecutions. Their review of the evidence led to a coroner's order to exhume the body of Mrs Katharine Armstrong from its grave in Cusop churchyard, where it had lain for ten months. Spilsbury was called in and travelled down to Hay by train via Hereford on 2 January 1922. He was met by the local police Superintendent, who escorted him to the graveside.

It was early evening on a winter's day and the scene was illuminated by hurricane lamps. The disinterred coffin was taken to an empty cottage nearby where it remained under police guard until the post-mortem examination the following day. Spilsbury was assisted by two local doctors in the grisly task of examining a long dead corpse. The body was removed from its oak coffin and placed on a trestle table from which drops of putrefied matter fell to the floor. Conditions such as these – poorly lit, badly ventilated and completely lacking in any washing facilities – were by no means unusual to pathologists of that era.

As he went about his task, Spilsbury's first observation was that the body was unusually well preserved and appeared to be undergoing mummification rather than putrefaction in the normal manner. He took various samples of fluid, tissue and organs from the body and put them into specimen jars for laboratory analysis. When the post-mortem examination had been completed, the body was left to be viewed by the coroner's jury and Spilsbury made a speedy return to London with his sixteen sample jars. He took them straight to St Mary's for the attention of John Webster, the senior Home Office analyst, and finished a long day by telephoning Willcox to discuss his initial findings.

The two men met on 12 February to review the scientific evidence, which included Webster's analyses. Large amounts of arsenic had been found in the liver and large intestine, the latter particularly indicating that poison had probably been administered within twenty-four hours of death. They appeared, together with John Webster, to give their evidence at the magistrates' court at Hay-on-Wye. The evidence for poisoning was overwhelming and Major Armstrong was committed to trial for the murder of his wife.

The trial at Hereford produced another powerful line-up of forensic talent. Mr Justice Darling presided and, as was traditional in poisoning cases, the prosecution was headed by the Attorney-General, Sir Ernest Pollock, with the defence in the hands of the redoubtable Sir Henry Curtis Bennett. Spilsbury and Willcox once again appeared together to present the medical evidence.

Major Armstrong was a small man who liked to cut a dash as a military figure with his heavy, waxed moustache and army officer's British warm overcoat. Weighing seven stone and standing five feet six inches tall, he was every bit the pocket soldier. He practised as a solicitor in Hay-on-Wye, which in the 1920s, was a small market town situated on the border of England and Wales. He was a well-known figure in the district, clerk to the local magistrates, a member of the local Territorial Army unit and a Freemason. This pillar of the community commanded respect by virtue of his position in the town's social pecking order but people sniggered behind his back at his posturing and because it was widely known that he was completely under the thumb of his overbearing wife.

Katharine Armstrong, a rather gaunt-looking lady, was prone to hypochondria and dosed herself with homeopathic medicines. She did not like people touching her, even accidentally, abhorred smoking, ran meals in her home according to a strict timetable and thought nothing of humiliating her husband in public. 'No wine for the Major' was her curt instruction to servants at local social functions.

Mrs Armstrong was taken ill in August 1920 and her doctor, Tom Hincks, arranged for her to be psychiatrically examined. As a result, she was certified insane and admitted to an asylum near Gloucester. She returned after five months and a nurse was brought in to look after her. During February 1921, her health declined and she suffered bouts of severe illness involving vomiting and diarrhoea. Her condition deteriorated rapidly and a stark entry in Major Armstrong's diary for 22 February read, 'K died'. She was buried without fuss, the doctor having certified cause of death as gastritis.

The Major inherited his wife's estate, amounting to some £2,000, and went on holiday. When he returned to Hay to what he doubtless imagined would be a new, trouble-free life, he encountered a problem in the shape of a rival young solicitor running a law practice from an office across the street from his own. The rival, a career-minded man by the name of Oswald Martin, was successful to the extent that some of Armstrong's clients had transferred their business to him. In August 1921, the two men clashed over a property deal in which Armstrong, acting for the purchaser, had delayed completion for over a year.

Martin began to put pressure on the Major to complete. After several weeks, Armstrong, having failed to respond, suddenly invited Martin to take tea with him at his house. On 26 October, Martin made his way to Armstrong's home at Cusop, just outside the town. They sat in the drawing room and drank tea and, at one stage, Armstrong offered his guest a buttered scone with the apology, 'Excuse fingers'. Various pleasantries ensued and in due course Martin took his leave. Late that same evening, he was taken violently ill with severe vomiting. The doctor diagnosed a bilious attack but the sick man's father-in-law who ran the town's pharmacy, thought otherwise.

Knowing of Martin's disagreement with Armstrong and being aware that he had taken tea with the Major, rang alarm bells with the chemist. He remembered that he had recently sold arsenic to Armstrong for the purpose of killing weeds. Apprehension grew stronger when Mrs Constance Martin recalled that a house guest had been taken ill after eating a chocolate from a box that had been delivered by the postman from an anonymous sender. It was agreed that the remaining chocolates and a sample of Oswald Martin's urine should be sent for analysis.

Oblivious to the fomenting suspicions about his intentions, Armstrong began to pester Martin with further invitations to tea. These were declined politely but firmly and, after six weeks of waiting, the results of the analysis were made known. Both the urine sample and the chocolates contained arsenic. The wheels of officialdom now moved swiftly and, on the last day of the year, an unsuspecting Major Armstrong, strongly protesting his innocence, was arrested. When he was searched, a packet of arsenic was found in his jacket pocket. This was to weigh heavily against him at his trial.

Armstrong was tried at the Shire Hall, Hereford in April 1922 before Mr Justice Darling; he pleaded 'Not Guilty'. The first expert witness for the prosecution was Spilsbury. He gave a report of his post-mortem findings and made it clear that a fatal dose of arsenic was ingested by Katharine Armstrong within twenty-four hours of her death. With the aid of a drawing depicting the human alimentary system, he pointed out the organs which had been subjected to analysis.

Sir Henry Curtis Bennett in his cross-examination of the pathologist tried to find an alternative to murder, such as a single, self-administered dose of arsenic on the part of a woman who had only recently been discharged from a mental institution. Try as he might, Sir Henry could not persuade Spilsbury to modify his views and the prosecution case strengthened when Webster and Willcox gave their evidence supporting his opinions. But Armstrong's final undoing was self-inflicted when he went into the witness box. During a six-hour ordeal he answered over 2,000 questions but the crucial exchange was with the judge. Darling asked him about the packet found in his pocket which contained enough arsenic to kill a human being and which he explained was for killing dandelions. Pressed to explain his laborious technique for dosing individual dandelions, his lame excuse was that it seemed 'the most convenient way'.

In his summing-up, Mr Justice Darling drew the attention of the jury to Spilsbury's evidence. He highlighted the pathologist's manner as much as his testimony. 'Do you remember Dr Spilsbury?' he asked. 'How he stood and the way in which he gave evidence? Did you ever see a witness who more thoroughly satisfied you that he was absolutely impartial, absolutely fair, absolutely indifferent as to whether his evidence told for the one side or the other?' Where he had merely impressed before, Spilsbury now seemed to have been gifted with something close to infallibility. In any event, the weight of the evidence against Armstrong, though circumstantial, was overwhelmingly in favour of guilt. He was convicted of murder and hanged at Gloucester Prison on 31 May 1922. In December of that year, Spilsbury received a letter from Mr Bonar Law, the Prime Minister, telling him that he had been awarded a knighthood.

Sir Bernard Spilsbury was soon in the news again, this time in connection with a case of murder and dismemberment, the solution of which many believed to be his greatest technical achievement. The crime committed by Patrick Mahon was discovered by chance. Mahon, a handsome man with charming ways, found married life somewhat dull and elected for the role of the philanderer. Worried about his unexplained absences from home, Mrs Mahon decided to search his clothes for some item, a letter perhaps, which might give a clue as to his actions. She found a cloakroom ticket issued at London's Waterloo station. A friend helped with her enquiries and they exchanged the ticket for a locked Gladstone bag. By prising open the ends of the bag, Mrs Mahon's companion, a former railway policeman, found some bloodstained female clothing and a knife. He immediately went to the police.

Mahon was picked up by the police when he appeared at Waterloo station to retrieve his bag. His explanation that the bag had been used for carrying dog meat immediately collapsed for it had already been established that the bloodstains were of human origin. Close interrogation of Mahon led the Sussex Police to a bungalow at Pevensey on the stretch of the Sussex coast known as The Crumbles. He had rented it in a false name at a charge of three and a half guineas a week. On 4 May 1924, Scotland Yard detectives accompanied by Spilsbury made an examination of the bungalow. What they found ranks as one of the most grisly murder cases in the history of British crime.

The rooms of the bungalow contained perfectly ordinary furniture and other articles and, at first glance, nothing appeared to be an immediate cause for concern. The casual observer might have thought it unusual, though, to find a saucepan full of liquid in the hearth of the living room fireplace while Spilsbury's trained eye took in a number of phenomena which, even at that early stage, began to tell him a story. There were grease splashes on the fender and bloodstains on the carpet. Worse was to come when various receptacles in that house of horrors were opened.

A hatbox in one of the bedrooms contained several pieces of flesh which had been sawn or cut up and a large trunk bearing the initials, EBK, contained four large pieces of a human body. A biscuit tin inside the trunk was filled with various internal organs. When the greasy scum on the surface of the liquid in the large saucepan was parted, a piece of boiled flesh floated to the surface. The ashes in the fireplace, when sieved, resulted in the discovery of bone fragments and so the trail of discovery continued. Protected by a long white apron and wearing rubber gloves, Spilsbury presided over the kitchen table which had been taken out into the garden. There, in bright May sunshine, he re-assembled the pieces of the body which had been brought to destruction in the bungalow. A contemporary press photograph depicted Spilsbury at work surrounded by watching police officers but the *disjecta membra* on the table had been air-brushed out of the picture in order not to offend public sensibilities.

Spilsbury spent eight hours at the bungalow and, at the end of the day, the remains returned with him to St Bartholomew's Hospital where he worked through the night to complete his examination. His report was a model of exactitude. He concluded that the body 'was that of an adult female of big build and fair hair. She was pregnant, in my opinion, at the time of death.' From the mass of rotting, boiled and burned remains, he had ascertained that no portion was duplicated and, therefore, that he was dealing with a single body. He later described the case as a 'jigsaw puzzle' but it was a puzzle from which the main piece, the head, was missing.

The EBK, whose initials appeared on the trunk in the bungalow, was Emily Beilby Kaye, a shorthand typist in her late thirties. It had been her misfortune to encounter Patrick Mahon with whom she fell in love despite the knowledge that he was already married. At the age of thirty-eight, she possibly thought that she was on the shelf and was overwhelmed by Mahon's winning ways. In March 1924, Emily told her friends she was engaged and that she planned to travel with her fiancé to South Africa where he had secured a job. Before embarking on this adventure, they decided to indulge in a 'love experiment', for which purpose Mahon rented the bungalow near Pevensey.

According to Mahon, the experiment went wrong when an argument broke out over his failure to obtain a passport allowing them to travel to South Africa as intended. He alleged that Emily attacked him, stumbling in the process, and fell heavily to the floor, fatally striking her head on the coal bucket. The knowledge that he had been systematically milking the poor, infatuated girl's savings and had purchased a knife and a tenon saw on his way down to Sussex suggested a different explanation. One of the first objects that had caught Spilsbury's eye when he entered the bungalow was the rusty tenon saw, it's teeth clogged with flesh – mute testimony to the violence that had been inflicted on Emily Kaye's body.

Patrick Mahon's tale of accidental death unravelled in court in the face of the pathologist's testimony. The coal bucket, a cauldron-shaped design standing on three legs, was a popular, cheaply made piece of hardware. It lacked the robustness of an inert object capable of causing a grievous wound to the head. As Spilsbury put it in his reply to defence counsel, J.D. Cassels, 'If that particular cauldron, filled with coal, were the one referred to, a sufficiently severe blow to produce such injury would have crumpled the cauldron.' In order that there should be no room for doubt on this question, prosecution counsel, Sir Henry Curtis Bennett, asked, 'In your opinion could Miss Kaye have received rapidly fatal injuries from falling on the coal cauldron?' Spilsbury's uncompromising reply was simply, 'No.'

An axe with a broken shaft was found in the bungalow and it was believed that this was the weapon which Mahon wielded with such force in striking Emily Kaye as to break the wooden handle. The victim's head was never found. Mahon's account was that he had burned the severed head in the fireplace at the bungalow and broken up the remains with a poker. No skull fragments were found in the ashes and doubt was cast on the possibility that an ordinary coal fire could have generated sufficient heat to destroy a head. In an experiment, reminiscent of that carried out by French experts investigating the Landru Case in 1921, Spilsbury succeeded in reducing a sheep's head to ashes in four hours. The stove in Landru's mansion at Gambais proved much more suitable for its task, consuming a sheep's head in a quarter of an hour!

While being questioned by defence counsel on the third day of the trial in humid July weather, Mahon was visibly shaken when a loud clap of thunder

sounded throughout the court building. If this was a signal from above, it probably endorsed the conclusion already being formed in the minds of the jury that
Mahon was a calculating and relentless murderer. He was duly found guilty and
sentenced to death. The 'Man of Prey', as the press called him, was executed at
Wandsworth Prison on 9 September 1924.

According to some, he was 'doubly hanged', for he was supposed to have used
his knowledge of the hangman's procedure to outwit the system. Despite being
hooded, he judged the moment when Albert Pierrepoint opened the trap and
jumped backwards onto the solid platform to avoid the drop. The result was that
his spine smashed against the edge of the woodwork with sufficient force to kill
him, followed by suspension at the end of the rope in the normal way which
broke his spine a second time.

But this was a matter on which Spilsbury, not for the last time, had the final
word, for he carried out the post-mortem examination of Mahon's body. It was
his first examination of an individual subjected to judicial hanging and was carried out with customary thoroughness. He noted that the spine was dislocated
between the fourth and fifth cervical vertebrae and that there was displacement
between the sixth and the seventh. He recorded no evidence of bruising which
would surely have been present if the hanging had occurred in the manner
described by Sir Henry Curtis Bennett's biographers.

Spilsbury's technical feat in re-assembling the fragmented remains of Patrick
Mahon's victim was acknowledged by Sir Archibald Bodkin, the Director of
Public Prosecutions, in a letter, when he wrote, '. . . I am sure that the learned
Judge and jury, Counsel, and last but not least myself, have deeply appreciated the
care and skill which you have brought to bear on this matter.'

Spilsbury's next big case was one in which his reputation, hitherto eulogised
almost as a matter of course, was seriously challenged. His protagonist was Dr
Robert Bronte, an Irishman who had come to England in 1922 to pursue his
medical career and took up an appointment as pathologist at Harrow Hospital in
Middlesex. He clashed with Spilsbury over the Thorne case in 1925 on a matter of
medical interpretation. Norman Thorne was a chicken farmer with poor prospects
who worked a poultry farm near Crowborough in Sussex. He lived in a converted
brooding hut on his plot of land and, although his circumstances were unappealing, if not squalid, he seemed attractive to Elsie Cameron, a London typist in her
early twenties, and they became engaged. Fearful that she had competition for his
affection, Elsie told Thorne that she was pregnant and reminded him that he had
promised to marry her. With a show of determination, she packed a bag and left
her home in London on 5 December 1924, intending to move in with her fiancé.

When the young woman failed to return home, her father contacted the police and, in due course, the trail led to Thorne's chicken farm. At first the police were satisfied with the answers he gave to their enquiries but, on a second visit, a search turned up Elsie's travel bag. Under questioning, Thorne said that he had found the girl hanging from a beam in his hut but was adamant that he had not killed her. He claimed that he decided to dispose of the body by cutting it into sections which he wrapped in sacking and buried in one of his chicken runs. Having cut off her head, he forced it into a tin box which he also buried.

Elsie Cameron's dismembered body was disinterred on 15 January 1925, nearly six weeks after she had disappeared. Spilsbury carried out the post-mortem examination after which the body was given a proper burial. By this time, Thorne was under arrest and charged with murder while his defence lawyers gathered their strength for a confrontation with Spilsbury. Their first decision was to retain the services of Dr Bronte as an expert witness. Declining to accept Spilsbury's findings, his opening move was to demand that the body of the recently buried Elsie be exhumed for a second post-mortem. This duly took place at the end of February, nearly three months after the time of death. Bronte reached different conclusions from those of Spilsbury and he was backed by six other medical witnesses mustered by Thorne's defence team.

The trial of Norman Thorne became an occasion for those who opposed Spilsbury's rise to eminence to challenge his opinion and perhaps overwhelm him by force of numbers. The battle lines were simply drawn out. The prosecution, led by the familiar courtroom figure of Sir Henry Curtis Bennett, and supported by Spilsbury was that Thorne had murdered his fiancée. J.D. Cassels, leading for the defence and with a small army of medical men by his side, argued that Elsie Cameron died of shock following an attempt at self-strangulation in the mistaken belief that she was pregnant. With Mr Justice Finlay presiding over his first murder trial at Lewes Assizes, the stage was set for controversy.

Spilsbury's expertise was to be tested in the interpretation of bruises, a field in which he was justifiably ranked as a leader. He gave it as his opinion that bruises found on the dead woman's body had been caused before death, one of which had resulted from a severe blow to the head. It was argued by the prosecution that Elsie Cameron had died from blows to the head inflicted by an Indian club. Arguing against this, the defence contended that the bruises had been caused accidentally when her limp, partially asphyxiated body fell to the floor during Thorne's attempt to save her life.

Spilsbury was adamant that death was caused by shock due to blows on the face and head. He discounted the possibility that the girl had attempted to hang herself, arguing that the laundry rope held to be the means of suspension would certainly have left an unmistakable mark on her neck. 'There was no such mark,' he said firmly. There were marks, though, on the dead girl's neck which Spilsbury discounted as having been caused by a ligature and which he described as natural folds or creases in the skin. Bronte's interpretation was different; he argued that these marks were the result of hanging and, as such, supported Thorne's account. Herein lay the main source of contention.

Spilsbury confirmed that he had made a thorough examination of the neck in view of the possibility that death might have been due to hanging. He had cut through a number of creases in the skin and found no area of haemorrhage suggesting that the tissues had been crushed or subjected to pressure by a rope. 'There was,' he said, 'no sign of any sort or kind of damage resulting from attempted hanging or actual hanging.' His judgement, therefore, was that it was not necessary to carry out any microscopic examination of tissues.

For his part, Bronte had insisted on taking tissues from the neck creases to be sectioned and prepared as microscope slides. Bearing in mind that decomposition of the body had advanced by a further month by the time he carried out the second post-mortem, Bronte had little hope of arguing a strong case from histological evidence. This did not prevent him from trying and he contended that his slides showed evidence of broken blood vessels in what he now termed 'grooves' in the neck, which were consistent with death by hanging. His case was that the creases (or grooves) in the neck were not natural folds in the skin as Spilsbury maintained, but the sort of marks that would be made by a cord.

Bronte also believed that his microscopic evidence disproved Spilsbury's opinion that there were no ruptured vessels in the neck with resultant escape of blood or extravasation into the tissues. The flamboyant Irishman was supported by a number of other medical men in court, one of whom described Spilsbury as very skilled but a trifle dogmatic. With his reputation under attack and, seemingly outnumbered, Spilsbury refused to capitulate. In a withering dismissal of Bronte's microscopical material, which he believed to be meaningless, he said of the slides, 'These might have been made anywhere, at any time. I cannot tell at all.'

Use of the word, 'infallible', in relation to Spilsbury's evidence seemed to be on everyone's lips at the conclusion of the trial. J.D. Cassels in his closing speech told the jury:

> What a tragedy of human justice it would be if the life of a man is to depend on the accuracy or infallibility of one individual. We can all admire attainment, take our hats off to ability, acknowledge the high position that a man has won in his sphere, but it is a long way to go to say that because that man says one thing, there can be no room for error.

Mr Justice Finlay told the jury, 'Sir Bernard Spilsbury would be the first to disclaim infallibility in matters of this sort,' but he added, 'his opinion is undoubtedly the very best that can be obtained.' Faced with the stark choice between murder by clubbing to death and suicide by hanging, the jury opted for murder. Despite the controversy over the medical evidence, the jury apparently found little difficulty in discharging their responsibility – they brought in a guilty verdict after retiring for only half an hour.

The controversy provoked by Thorne's trial did not stop at the verdict. The case was taken to appeal and Cassels asked the Lord Chief Justice to refer the medical evidence to an independent assessor as provided for by a 1907 amendment to the Criminal Appeal Act. After due consideration, this request was turned down on the grounds that there was no case for suggesting the jury had not understood the evidence put before them. The appeal was rejected and Norman Thorne was executed at Wandsworth Prison on 22 April 1925. Police searches at Thorne's chicken farm provided two interesting footnotes to the case. The dust on the crossbeam in the roof of his hut from which he claimed to have found Elsie Cameron hanging was said to be undisturbed and, among his belongings, were found newspaper cuttings reporting the trial of Patrick Mahon a few months before.

Criticism of Spilsbury continued after the trial had been concluded. The suggestion that the great man might have erred became something of a running battle for years and Dr Bronte appeared from time-to-time as protagonist for the critics. The *Law Journal* criticised the Appeal Court's decision to reject Thorne's appeal and said that the man had been 'condemned by a tribunal which was not capable of forming a first-hand judgement, but followed the man with the biggest name.' This was a sad condemnation of the twelve jurors who had reached a unanimous verdict.

An anonymous correspondent in one of the daily newspapers, calling himself a 'medico-legal expert', expressed his concern over Spilsbury's apparently infallible status. 'For some reason or other', he wrote, 'Sir Bernard Spilsbury has now arrived at a position where his utterances in the witness box commonly receive unquestioning acceptance from judge, counsel and jury.' The knives were out and it would later become fashionable to say that Spilsbury's talents were too highly regarded. The man himself appeared untouched by the whole business and privately expressed his dislike for what he believed were unprofessional and slapdash methods used by some of his opponents, including Bronte, for whom he reserved the epithet, 'that man'.

While Spilsbury was dodging the arrows of professional jealousy, other bright stars in the pathology firmament were beginning to rise. Sydney Smith was working in Egypt and developing the science of firearms evidence following the murder of Sir Lee Stack in 1924, John Glaister was in general practice in Glasgow but increasingly helping with police work, and Francis Camps was studying for his final medical examinations at Guy's Hospital Medical School. In due course, Spilsbury would clash with both Smith and Glaister while Camps would turn out to be something of a maverick in a similar mould to Bronte.

Spilsbury's biographers addressed a note, 'to those who know a pathologist only as an expert witness in criminal cases'. They pointed out that murder cases which made big newspaper headlines and caught the public imagination were, in reality, only a small part of the workload. Although he was rarely out of the news, Spilsbury did not spare himself in the efforts he devoted to the routine work required by coroners' courts. H.R. Oswald, senior coroner of the County of London, writing in his memoirs in 1938, spoke of making Spilsbury's acquaintance twenty years earlier when he asked the Home Office to send him a specialist to deal with the murder of a girl on Eltham Common. 'They sent me Mr Spilsbury,' he wrote, and continued, 'he was so precise, skilful and exact in giving his evidence that I was impressed, and used constantly, after that, to ask him to investigate any important case that came through my Courts, and other Coroners did the same.' Ingleby Oddie, coroner for Central London, also made good use of Spilsbury's services as did Bentley Purchase, coroner for North London.

Spilsbury's meticulous attention to detail and his willing acceptance of a heavy workload was commented on by the coroners for whom he worked. There were some who thought he was unnecessarily zealous at times and, consequently, at fault for not maintaining a proper perspective. Even where the cause of death was demonstrably straightforward, he could not resist the temptation to extend a post-mortem examination and take samples for his own interest. His friend, William Willcox, told his son, 'Spilsbury is a fool: he'll kill himself with work done for nothing.' Sadly, the truth of this was borne out in subsequent events, although, arguably, it was not for nothing.

He brought the same professional standards of competence to his routine work as he did to that which assumed national importance. Sometimes, he confounded his friends with his inflexible attitude, as on the occasion he was asked by Sir Walter Schroder, one of the London coroners, to take a second look at a body; 'I never do that,' was the reply.

At his peak, Spilsbury was carrying out 1,000 post-mortem examinations a year, the details of many of them ending up on his record cards. The habits of the loner which had been evident during his student days stayed with him during his professional career. He did not use a secretary and preferred to write his reports by hand, often in the grim surroundings of a mortuary while details were still fresh in his mind. He was a familiar and regular visitor at many of London's mortuaries whose attendants respected him for his courtesy and habit of tipping.

He also spent a great deal of what others would have regarded as leisure time in his laboratory at home where he had facilities for sectioning and microscopy.

Many hours of midnight oil were burnt in the service of forensic pathology and in the satisfaction of the singular motivation which drove him on. He had a sense of his own greatness which surfaced in the professional encounters engineered by those who wished to bring him down and which occasionally emerged in conversational exchanges.

Most of Spilsbury's work kept him in London and, unlike Smith and Glaister, he did not seek experience abroad. London's courts, with occasional excursion to the county assizes, were his parish but it was the one per cent of his case load constituting murder enquiries which continued to seize the headlines. In February 1927, he made one of his rare sorties out of London when he took part in a controversial trial in Edinburgh. What was even more unusual was that he appeared as an expert witness for the defence. The case concerned John Merrett who was charged with matricide, which ranks as one of the least practised forms of murder. By a strange coincidence, Spilsbury was to be involved in two cases of matricide in the space of three years.

In Edinburgh's High Court of Justiciary, the man accused of murder, John Donald Merrett, was a teenager who had come to England with his mother from New Zealand. In 1926, he was a non-resident student at Edinburgh University and lived with his mother in a furnished flat where a daily maid attended to the routine domestic work. Young Merrett's passion, however, was more for girls than learning, with the consequence that he ducked lectures and quickly consumed his allowance of ten shillings a week.

In March 1926, an apparently tranquil domestic scene in the Merrett household was shattered by the sound of a gunshot. Mrs Bertha Merrett had been writing letters at her bureau in the sitting room. Her son was sitting in a chair reading and the maid was working in the kitchen. Startled by the noise, the maid rushed into the sitting room to be met by Merrett, who exclaimed, 'My mother has shot herself.' Mrs Merrett lay on the floor bleeding from a head wound and an automatic pistol lay on the bureau. She was still alive when taken to Edinburgh Royal Infirmary where she lingered in a semi-conscious state for two weeks.

She died on 1 April from meningitis but not before she had spoken about her recollections of what had taken place. She recalled that her son was being a nuisance by interrupting her while she was writing letters and that she told him to go away and stop annoying her. She had no idea of what precisely happened next although she seemed surprised that a firearm was involved. Mrs Merrett was accorded a suicide's burial.

The dead woman's estate was left in trust for her son to inherit when he was twenty-five years old. In the meantime, in order to finance his playboy lifestyle, he borrowed money from his relatives. In the ensuing months, it became clear that during the last months of his mother's life he had been milking her bank accounts by forging cheques. Police enquiries followed and, nine months after the shooting incident, eighteen-year-old Merrett was charged with both murder and forgery.

The trial for murder in Edinburgh brought together a number of leading figures from the medico-legal world. Two stalwarts from the forensic medicine scene in Scotland were called by the prosecution; Professor Harvey Littlejohn from Edinburgh and Professor John Glaister senior from Glasgow. The two professors were advised by Sir Sydney Smith, an outspoken critic of Spilsbury, who was on holiday in Edinburgh at the time, and assisted by Dr John Glaister. Spilsbury, on this occasion appearing for the defence, was partnered by Robert Churchill, the London gun expert with whom he had worked before.

The point to be settled was whether the shot that killed Mrs Merrett had been fired accidentally, deliberately to commit suicide, or as an act of murder. Doctors who had examined the injured woman when she was admitted to the infirmary observed no signs of blackening or tattooing around the wound in her right ear where the bullet had entered. Such evidence would be expected in a case of suicide when it is usual for the weapon to be held close to, or in contact with, the skin. It was reported that a great deal of blood had been washed away from the wound using water-soaked swabs and that the subsequent examination for powder tattooing was only made by means of the naked eye.

The absence of tattooing made it difficult to argue forcibly in favour of suicide. The experts called by the prosecution were inclined at first to the view that the shooting was 'consistent with suicide' but then changed their minds. This followed consultation with Sydney Smith, a man of acknowledged expertise in the field of forensic ballistics and the assessment of gunshot wounds, who said, 'It looks to me like murder.' He advised Littlejohn and Glaister to carry out a few tests with the weapon involved in the shooting to establish its discharge characteristics.

The Spanish-made .25 automatic was used to fire ammunition of the same manufacture as that used in the fatal shooting into paper targets at distances ranging from half an inch to twelve inches. At six inches, all signs of powder blackening around the bullet hole had disappeared, although a few tattoo spots were visible without the use of magnification. Aided by Professor Glaister, further experiments were carried out using an amputated limb obtained from a hospital operating theatre. The conclusion drawn in Glaister's report was that while not entirely ruling out the possibility of a self-inflicted wound, he believed it was an improbable explanation. In other words, he opted for murder.

Spilsbury and Churchill carried out their own experiments using an identical firearm and a different batch of ammunition. The gunsmith advised that the absence of scorching or blackening around the wound was not significant. In the first place, superficial blackening might have been washed away by the flow of blood and, secondly, the particular ammunition which had caused the fatal injury employed smokeless flake powder which caused less discoloration than gunpowder.

Not satisfied with arguments unsupported by experiment, and as Churchill told him that firing at paper targets produced unrealistic results, Spilsbury also went in search of a supply of amputated limbs. Test firings into dead flesh at various distances proved to their satisfaction that flake powder did not tattoo the skin and that traces of blackening were only superficial. Consequently, their opinion was that in the circumstances of the shooting, suicide was a distinct possibility.

The prosecution's experts did not give the impression that they were entirely convinced by their own arguments and Professor Glaister, in particular, resorted frequently to the use of the word 'probable' to qualify his statements. Defence counsel, Craigie Aitchison, drew out this hesitation in cross-examination and he also distinguished himself when Spilsbury was called by addressing his expert as 'Saint Bernard'. Spilsbury's contribution in support of Robert Churchill's testimony was given with customary precision. In essence, his opinion was that he had found nothing that was inconsistent with the notion of suicide. On the vital question regarding the significance of powder blackening around the wound, he felt that no firm conclusion could be drawn in circumstances where there had been considerable bleeding and subsequent cleaning of the wound.

The jury returned a verdict of Not Proven on the murder charge but found Merrett guilty of forgery. He was sentenced to one year's imprisonment. After serving his sentence, he married a teenage girl, inherited £50,000 and changed his name to Chesney. It was as Ronald Chesney that in 1954 he murdered his wife and mother-in-law and finally shot himself. Spilsbury was dead himself by then but his part in helping Merrett to retain his freedom in Edinburgh twenty-seven years earlier did not go unremarked. Indeed Sir Sydney Smith demonstrated some venom when he wrote in his memoirs, 'The slackness of the police and the credit given to the misleading evidence of Spilsbury and Churchill, who had made a mistake and were too stubborn to admit it, allowed Merrett to live – and to kill again.' Thus, Spilsbury's excursion into the realm of the defence expert was pursued by controversy.

A few weeks after the case against Merrett was found controversially Not Proven, Spilsbury was involved in an enquiry that was merely sensational – it concerned a trunk deposited at the luggage office at Charing Cross railway station in London. It had been left on 6 May 1927 and was soon the subject of attention on account of the awful stench which it emitted. The trunk was opened under police supervision and it was not long before Spilsbury had the task of making a close examination of its contents.

The putrefying remains in the trunk proved to be the dismembered body of a woman. From bruises and other indications, Spilsbury was able to ascertain that the woman, whose identity was unknown, had been asphyxiated. Articles of clothing in the trunk carried laundry marks and one bore a tab with the name, 'P. Holt', printed on it. The garments were traced to an address in Chelsea and the body in the trunk was identified within twenty-four hours as that of Minnie Bonati, a married Italian lady of promiscuous inclinations who had been working as a cook.

Within a week, a taxi driver had come forward to report that on 6 May he had been hired by a man who lived in Rochester Row to drive him to Charing Cross railway station. He easily remembered the incident as his fare needed assistance to move a heavy trunk. A search of the premises resulted in the discovery that an estate agent by the name of John Robinson, who rented a furnished room in the building, was absent. Robinson was apprehended in London on 19 May and, after a false start, when neither the taxi driver nor the porter at Charing Cross left luggage office could positively identify him, he gave himself away during questioning.

Robinson's story was that he had met Mrs Bonati and taken her back to his office. There, she had demanded money and became aggressive. She hit out at him and, in the resulting scuffle, he retaliated and she fell, dazed, to the floor. Later, he found that she was dead and, faced with disposing of her body, decided on dismemberment. By an extraordinary coincidence or piece of copycat planning, Robinson went in search of a suitable knife and found what he wanted at the shop in Victoria Street where, three years previously, Patrick Mahon had bought his implements of destruction. He then obtained a trunk in Brixton and, under the very noses of the officers of Rochester Row police station, had it transported with its grim contents to Charing Cross.

Robinson's thin story line was readily disproved in court and his trial for murder lasted only two days. The medical evidence proved conclusively that the bruises on Bonati's body were not the result of a fall but of a succession of blows followed by asphyxiation. Asked how the bruises had been caused, Spilsbury's reply was characteristically direct; 'Most of them were caused by direct violence,' he said. In what must have been seen as virtually a lost cause by the defence, the indefatigable Dr Bronte was produced to repute Spilsbury's findings and lend weight to the accused man's account of an accidental death. His arguments proved equally thin and Robinson was found guilty.

It was not long before the two pathologists were again pitched into the arena as opponents. Between April 1928 and March 1929, three members of the same family in Croydon died of arsenical poisoning. Edmund Creighton Duff was a former Colonial civil servant who had retired to Surrey in the same community as his mother-in-law, Violet Sydney, a barrister's widow who lived with her unmarried daughter, Vera. Fifty-nine-year-old Duff died at his home on 27 April 1928 after a brief illness. The family doctor was puzzled by his symptoms but suspected food poisoning. At the post-mortem, Dr Robert Bronte took samples of the body organs for analysis but found no evidence of poisoning. Death from natural causes was duly confirmed.

In February 1929, Vera Sydney was taken ill with severe vomiting and died within forty-eight hours; gastric influenza was diagnosed. Three weeks later, her mother, Violet Sydney, still grieving the loss of her daughter, was herself taken ill with similar symptoms. The family doctor diagnosed food poisoning. Mrs Sydney's son, Thomas, who also lived in Croydon, perhaps anxious about his own well-being, sought further medical advice. Bacteriological tests on the dead women proved inconclusive and the family did not feel inclined to pursue the matter any further. Yet the occurrence of two sudden deaths in the same household within such a short period excited attention in official circles and the Home Office ordered an enquiry.

The bodies of Vera and Violet Sydney were exhumed from their graves at Croydon Cemetery on 22 March 1929 and Spilsbury carried out the post-mortem examinations. The most notable and immediate observation was one that had echoes of the Armstrong case. After six weeks' burial, the body of Vera Sydney appeared to be remarkably well-preserved. Inflammation of the stomach and urinary tract in both sets of remains, considered in light of the symptoms the women had experienced, suggested arsenical poisoning.

Confirmation of this tentative diagnosis came from analyses carried out by Dr John Ryffel, one of the Home Office analysts. He found 1.48 grains of arsenic in Vera Sydney's body and 3.48 grains in that of Violet Sydney. Arsenic present in her hair and nails indicated that the older woman had been ingesting the poison over a considerable period. Traces of arsenic found in the tonic medicine prescribed by her family doctor indicated the vehicle by which she had probably been poisoned.

Attention now focused on Edmund Duff whose remains had been interred for just over a year. Despite the fact that analyses carried out at the time had proved negative for traces of poison, an exhumation order was granted. On 18 May 1929, notebook in hand, Spilsbury appeared at the graveside at Queen's Road Cemetery and was soon joined by Dr Gerald Roche Lynch, Senior Official Analyst at the Home Office. Spilsbury carried out the post-mortem in the presence of the analysts, Dr Bronte and the Duff family's doctor. The experts made their reports and, after high-level legal consultation, a second inquest was ordered in respect of the death of Edmund Duff. Meanwhile, the inquest on Vera Sydney was still proceeding. The inquests on the three deceased members of the Duff and Sydney families were held separately and, with various adjournments, dragged on for five months. The coroner, who declined to accept advice from the Director of Public Prosecutions to hold the inquests together, was heavily criticised for creating confusion. And, when it came to the inquest on Duff, confusion indeed reigned supreme.

Spilsbury related the facts of the post-mortem examination that he had carried out, noting that the body bore the marks of the incisions made during the first such examination. He also pointed out that most of the organs were missing. The inflamed condition of the intestines left in the body suggested some form of gastro-intestinal irritation and this was consistent with the symptoms suffered by the patient during his illness. The well-preserved condition of the body was also remarked on. Dr Roche Lynch then gave the results of the analyses he had carried out on the organ and tissue samples which Spilsbury had removed from the corpse. He had calculated there was a total of 0.815 grains of arsenic in the tissues. Taking all the circumstances into account, he concluded that Edmund Duff had died of acute arsenical poisoning.

This had the effect of putting Bronte on the spot because the possibility of arsenical poisoning had not featured in his report of the first post-mortem examination. He had, though, jotted down the letters 'AS', signifying arsenic, on the carbon copy of his report, denoting that he had considered the possibility. While this may have appeared to be an afterthought, worse was to come when it seemed that part of another body had become mixed up with the organs removed from Duff. Bronte had no answer for this except to suggest that someone had interfered with the sealed specimen jars. At any rate, it was confirmed that tests on the organs purporting to be those of Edmund Duff had been carried out at the London Hospital Medical School, with negative results for arsenic. Bronte agreed that his original finding of death from natural causes was wrong and confirmed that he now believed Duff had died from arsenical poisoning.

Spilsbury's opinion was that Duff had ingested a fatal dose of arsenic within twenty-four hours of death. The likely vehicle seemed to be the bottled beer he had drunk with his supper after returning home from a fishing holiday. The chicken he had consumed was ruled out because his wife had eaten the same meal and not been unwell. Sir Bernard was closely questioned by William Fearnley-Whittingstall, the young barrister representing the Duff and Sydney families. The twenty-six-year-old advocate gave the pathologist a hard time in what was described as a brilliant piece of advocacy. He attacked the basis of Spilsbury's opinion that Duff took in the arsenic with his beer. They sparred over the pros and cons of the chicken as the purveyor of the poison, discussed the intricacies of digestion and debated the effect that Duff's feverish cold might have had on events. At the end of it all, Spilsbury remained adamant that the arsenic had been ingested via the beer. This, of course, cast suspicion on the family or, at least, on someone close.

The coroner's jury concluded that Edmund Duff had died from arsenical poisoning, wilfully administered by some person or persons unknown. A similar verdict had been reached at the inquest into the death of Vera Sydney, but in the case of her mother, Violet, the jury was unable to decide whether she had been murdered or had committed suicide, although they were sure that arsenical poisoning was the cause of her death. In a full account of the Croydon poisonings, written in 1975, Richard Whittington-Egan concluded that the murders, which had thus far remained unsolved, were committed by Grace Duff, Edmund's wife, who hated her spouse and wanted to eliminate him. According to this thesis, she poisoned Violet and Vera Sydney simply for gain.

In the winter of 1929, Spilsbury featured in his second case of matricide and headed once more for a confrontation with Bronte. On 23 October, a fire at the Metropole Hotel in Margate appeared to have claimed the life of an elderly resident. The fire alarm was raised by Sidney Fox, who was staying at the hotel with his mother, and fellow residents dragged the semi-conscious old lady from her smoke-filled room. Medical assistance was sent for but Rosaline Fox was already dead by the time the doctor arrived. Her son was distraught and between sobs of 'My Mummy, my Mummy,' told the hotel manager, 'She is all I have in the world.' The inquest on Mrs Fox concluded with a verdict of death by misadventure. She was buried in Norfolk and on the day of her funeral, her son travelled to Norwich to make a claim on her life insurance policy. The insurance company was immediately suspicious and a wire was sent to its head office carrying the message, 'Very muddy water in this business.'

Sidney Fox was arrested on a charge of fraudulent dealing, while, behind the scenes, the wheels turned very quickly indeed. Scotland Yard detectives were called in and Spilsbury was alerted. On 9 November, the pathologist was at the graveside of Mrs Fox, supervising the exhumation of her body. A post-mortem examination followed and, thus, the die was cast for another medico-legal controversy.

The circumstances of Mrs Fox's death, coupled with the behaviour of her son, and his established reputation as a fraudster, had provoked suspicion of murder. The initial focus of attention had been the room in which the victim was found and, in particular, the chair which appeared to have been the centre of the fire. The carpet had been burnt underneath the chair and the burning upholstery of the furniture seemed to have been the source of the dense smoke which filled the room. It was strange, therefore, that Spilsbury found no trace of carbon monoxide in the blood nor in the sooty deposits usually found in the air passages when a person breathes in smoke. Absence of such evidence suggested that the victim was already dead and that a cause other than the fire should be sought. It was Spilsbury's task to search for that cause and he established it, at least to his satisfaction, when he discovered a bruise at the back of Mrs Fox's throat. His conclusion was that she had been strangled.

Sidney Fox was eventually trapped by the thoroughness of two persons – the undertaker, who hermetically sealed the coffin with putty, and Spilsbury, whose eagle eye spotted a bruise on tissues which would rapidly decompose when exposed to the air. When the case came to trial, the pathologist was confronted by familiar adversaries, J.D. Cassels, who defended Fox on the charge of murder, and, of course, Dr Bronte. For the first time too, he also faced a fellow pathologist of considerable eminence and reputation, in the presence of Professor Sydney Smith who supported the defence.

The prosecution, led by the Attorney-General, Sir William Jowitt, with the aid of Margate Fire Brigade, proved fairly convincingly that a fire had been deliberately started in Mrs Fox's hotel room. There was a bottle of petrol in the room which Fox claimed he used to clean his clothes. It was known that Mrs Fox had been drinking port bought by her son and the alcohol found in her body suggested that she may well have been asleep when her demise occurred. But how did she die?

Spilsbury was convinced that she had not died of suffocation – the lack of sooty deposits in the air passages effectively ruled that out. His contention that Mrs Fox had been strangled was based on his discovery of a large, recent bruise at the back of the larynx. He demonstrated its position to the court by means of an anatomical model of the human mouth and throat. The bruise was the result of mechanical violence which tore open some of the small blood vessels, indicating, as he said, 'the conclusions to which I finally came, that death was due to strangulation.' Questioned about the condition of the hyoid bone which is situated in the larynx and becomes brittle in elderly people, the pathologist confirmed that it had not been broken in this instance. He acknowledged that the hyoid frequently was broken in cases of manual strangulation but, equally, he knew of many cases where this was not so.

The trouble with the bruise on the larynx was its somewhat ephemeral existence. After the organ had been removed from the body which had lain in its airtight coffin, the tissues rapidly putrefied when exposed to the atmosphere, obscuring the bruise and making its existence impossible to demonstrate. Thus, by the time Bronte came to examine the larynx, there was no bruise to be seen. The absence of such an injury that could be shown as a physical entity, made it easier for the defence to argue that Mrs Fox had died of heart failure. But, Spilsbury's word that he had seen it was sufficient to make it a matter of contention.

Short of accusing his opponent of fabricating evidence, all that Bronte could say was, 'It was not there when I saw the larynx.' Sir Bernard would not be moved from his position and his reply to Cassels's question on the matter put it beyond further debate; 'It was a bruise and nothing else. There are no two opinions about it'. As Sydney Smith put it in his autobiography, 'The oracle had spoken. There was nothing more to be said.'

Smith later mentioned an incident in Spilsbury's laboratory at University College Hospital when he and Bronte were shown the larynx preserved in formalin. 'I can't see any sign of a bruise, Spilsbury,' said Smith with nodding approval from Bronte. 'No, you can't see it now,' replied Spilsbury, 'but it was there when I exhumed the body.' Smith recorded that Spilsbury listened attentively and politely to his arguments but added, 'Had I known him then as well as I came to later, I would have realised why I was wasting my time. He could not change his opinion now because he had already given it.'

Sidney Fox, who, in a devastating admission in court, said that he had closed the door to his mother's room after discovering the fire and running for help, was found guilty of murder. He was a greedy little man and a poseur of the type that it has been said would sell their own grandmother. In his case, he throttled his mother for the insurance money and his guilt was perhaps so borne in on him that he did not bother to appeal against his conviction.

Thus began the decade of the 1930s, which produced more headline-snatching cases and rumbles of violence to come. One of Spilsbury's first cases in the new decade was the sensational 'Blazing Car Murder'. Appropriately enough, the incident occurred on Guy Fawkes Night in November 1930, when two youths returning from a bonfire night dance in Northampton, saw a burning car on the road near Hardingstone. There was a person in the car but rescue was out of the question because the blaze was too fierce.

The following day, the police decided to remove the charred corpse from the vehicle and away from public curiosity. The burnt-out wreckage of the car was pushed off the road to allow normal traffic to proceed without hindrance. These actions would later be heavily criticised. The owner of the car was traced by means of its still intact registration number, to Alfred Arthur Rouse, a commercial traveller, who lived in north London. But the identity of the person incinerated in the blaze remained uncertain.

Following reports of the burning car incident in the newspapers, Rouse returned to London from Wales where he had been visiting his girlfriend, and was greeted by detectives. The two young men who had arrived at the scene of the blaze in Hardingstone Lane, identified him as the person who had startled them by suddenly materialising out of the smoke. Rouse told the police that while travelling to Leicester on his firm's business, he stopped on the Great North Road to give a lift to a man who said he wanted to travel to the Midlands.

He explained that, first, he lost his way and then ran out of petrol. Before walking a short distance down the road in order to relieve himself, he asked his travelling companion to fill the car's fuel tank from a spare can of petrol which he provided. At this point, Rouse said he noticed a big flame and realised that the car was on fire. He rushed towards the blaze and tried to free the man who was trapped inside the vehicle but was beaten back by the ferocity of the flames. Then, in his statement to the police, he said, 'I lost my head.'

The fire had been tremendously fierce and the destruction wrought on the unfortunate individual caught inside the car was swift. The lower parts of his legs had been burned away as had the hands and forearms. There was massive destruction of the chest and abdomen and the head had burst in the intense heat. The body was never identified and even its gender was in doubt. Spilsbury, nevertheless recorded the victim as male, probably aged about thirty. A wooden mallet found near the burnt-out car was acknowledged by Rouse as belonging to him; he said he used it to loosen the cap on the petrol can. Several hairs on the mallet, judged by the pathologist to be of human origin, added weight to the conjecture that it had been used as a weapon of assault, if not murder.

Rouse was tried for murder at Northampton Assizes when the task of establishing how the victim of the blazing car met his death was made difficult by the unprofessional handling of vital evidence during the early stages of the police investigation. The charred body had been moved from the vehicle without first making *in situ* drawings or taking photographs. Reconstruction of the scene depended on eyewitness accounts, from which it appeared that the body had been lying face down across the two front seats with one leg extended through the open nearside door. In answer to questions put by Norman Birkett, who led for the prosecution, Spilsbury gave it as his belief that the victim was unconscious when the fire started and that, in all probability, the nearside door was open at the time. This certainly put Rouse's alleged rescue attempt into perspective.

Another unsatisfactory aspect of the investigation had been the way in which the wrecked car had been pushed to the side of the road and left unattended. In due course, the car was taken to Angel Lane police station where it was examined by Colonel Buckle, an experienced fire assessor, who found that the petrol union joint situated under the fuel tank behind the dashboard was loose by a full turn and there was evidence that the carburettor had been tampered with. The implications were obvious to the jury. Even the defence's medical witness agreed that it looked as if an unconscious man had been thrown into the car and the sinister interpretation of what followed was that the inert figure was dowsed with petrol and a fuel trail laid along the road which was then ignited from a safe distance.

Rouse, a salesman whose job enabled him to travel around the country to attend to what he liked to call his harem, was found guilty and sentenced to death. He went to appeal on the grounds that the prosecution should have proved motive, especially in a case where the victim was unidentified. The appeal failed and Rouse was hanged on 10 March 1931. His confession was published a month later in the *Daily Sketch*. At least, on this occasion, Spilsbury's critics had no grounds to contest his findings. As his biographers observed, 'this time no one grumbled – not even *The Law Journal*.'

In the course of a long career, a forensic pathologist may expect, sooner or later, to encounter every type of case. This was certainly true for Spilsbury and providence seemed inclined to serve him double helpings of the more unusual cases. He had already worked on two matricides when, in 1934, he was presented with a pair of trunk murders.

The Brighton Trunk Crimes became one of the sensations of the 1930s and, not least, because, for a long while, both were without satisfactory conclusion. In June 1934, a plywood trunk was deposited at the cloakroom in Brighton railway station. Some days later, the unsavoury smell pervading the atmosphere was traced to the box and the police were called. The offensive smell arose from the decaying female torso, minus head and legs, which was the trunk's principal contents. As the result of a nationwide alert to railway left luggage offices, a suspicious-looking suitcase was pinpointed at Kings Cross station in London. It contained what proved to be the legs belonging to the Brighton torso.

In the popular newspaper reporting of the day, it was noted that, 'Spilsbury was called in'. He confirmed the relationship between the two discoveries of body parts by showing that the saw cuts on the thigh bones of the legs matched the stumps on the torso. The remains were those of a pregnant woman aged about twenty-five who appeared well-nourished and free from disease. Cause of death was not apparent and Spilsbury reported that dismemberment had been carried out after death. He could only conjecture at the likely cause of death which, in the absence of capillary haemorrhages and draining of blood from the heart, tended to rule out strangulation and shooting. In all probability, fatal violence had been inflicted on the woman's head which was subsequently severed from the body and, together with the arms and hands, remained missing.

Police began the painstaking routine of checking missing persons files and following up the slenderest of clues. Part of the investigation involved house-to-house enquiries and it was a procedure which turned up the second Brighton Trunk Crime. Number 52 Kemp Street, near the railway station, was empty and locked up when a search was made of the district. When the house was entered on

13 July, the offensive smell which caused the searchers to gag, was traced to a large, locked trunk in one of the rooms. Tightly packed into its confined space was the body of a woman, decomposing but otherwise intact. Once again, Spilsbury was called in and he repeated the journey he had made to Brighton a month before in order to examine the victim of this second trunk crime.

On this occasion, the cause of death was readily apparent and was recorded on the pathologist's case card as shock resulting from a depressed fracture of the skull. A violent blow had broken a piece of bone out of the skull and forced it down onto the brain. The victim, aged about forty, wore a wedding ring and some of her clothes had been packed in the trunk with the body. Her identity was quickly established as Violette Kaye, a dancer, whose real name was Violet Saunders, and who had been missing since May. She had been considered, but ruled out of the investigation into Trunk Crime No. 1, on account of her age.

Her companion, a supposed Italian waiter named as Tony Mancini, was now urgently sought after by the police. He was apprehended in Blackheath on 18 July and taken to Brighton for questioning. Mancini's real name was Lois England and, despite his Italian appearance, he was English. He was a petty crook and lived off Violette Kaye's earnings from prostitution. In answer to the charge that he had killed her, he said, 'I am quite innocent, except for the fact that I kept the body hidden.'

Mancini was tried for murder and had the benefit of being defended by Norman Birkett, a man as acclaimed in his forensic field as Spilsbury was in his. The prosecution case was that Violette Kaye had been killed by a blow from a weapon such as a hammer which had been found in the cellar of the house in Park Crescent where she lived with Mancini. Evidence was given of an argument between them which indicated a possible motive. Mancini's story was that he had returned to the flat on the evening of 10 May to find Violette lying on the bed amid bloodstained sheets. He assumed that she had been killed by one of her customers. To explain his subsequent actions, Mancini said that because of his record, he knew the police would not believe him if he reported what he had found.

He decided therefore to hide the body by concealing it in a trunk which he bought for seven shillings and sixpence from a stall at Brighton market. When he moved house, claiming that he had left Violette because she nagged him, he took her remains in the trunk with him.

When he entered the witness box to give his evidence, Spilsbury had with him a skull and the piece of bone from Violette Kaye's head so that he could demonstrate the violent effect of the blow which killed her. Birkett immediately objected to this, claiming that the defence had not been advised about this particular exhibit. 'For a piece of bone which has been in existence all this time to be produced on the third day of the trial does put the defence in some difficulty,' he complained.

'I do not think it would take anyone long to examine it and come to conclusions,' countered Spilsbury.

Birkett then tried to persuade the pathologist that a fall down the basement steps at Park Crescent, resulting in collision with the iron rail at the bottom, could have produced a similar fracture.

'I think it impossible,' was Spilsbury's brief but polite response. Counsel decided to press the matter.

'Are you telling the members of the jury that if someone fell down that flight and came upon the stone ledge, he would not get a depressed fracture?'

'He would not get *this* fracture,' Spilsbury answered emphatically.

Mancini went into the witness box and, asked by the judge why he had not fetched the police after discovering the body, he replied, 'I considered that a man who had been convicted never gets a fair and square deal from the police'. Whether out of sympathy for the underdog or, perhaps, swayed by the doubts about motive and cause of death put forward by Birkett, the jury found Mancini 'Not Guilty'.

The outcome was a triumph for Birkett and his performance was described as ranking 'as one of the great defences in the annals of legal records'. But, in the stranger-than-fiction climate which often prevails in the world of crime, Birkett's success was undermined by his client who, many years later, confessed to murdering Violette Kaye. Mancini's story was published in the *News of the World* in November 1976, in the knowledge that he could not be tried again for a crime of which he had been acquitted.

In 1978, he elaborated on his confession and this was published in an account of the case in *Perfect Murder*, written by Bernard Taylor and Stephen Knight in 1987. In the end, Spilsbury was right about the fracture not being caused by falling down the basement steps but neither was it caused by a hammer blow. According to Mancini, he knocked Violette Kaye to the floor during an argument and, in a blind rage, smashed her head against the fireplace fender. Thus, the second of the two Brighton trunk murders which had remained officially solved during Spilsbury's lifetime, was finally resolved. The first one remains a mystery and the victim was never identified.

While Spilsbury had been exercised by the murders in Brighton, Keith Simpson was just starting out on his career. As a young demonstrator in pathology at Guy's Hospital in 1934, Simpson prospered from some of the antagonistic feelings that were directed at Spilsbury, as a result of which the Southwark coroner, Douglas Cowburn, declined to give his work to Sir Bernard. It was a perfect example of the jealousy and small-mindedness which ran as a consistent thread through otherwise impeccable professional lives.

The lack of a few more post-mortem examinations would hardly have bothered Spilsbury, who was overworked anyway, and young Dr Simpson was, no doubt, just as pleased to be advancing in his chosen career. Cases in profusion came to Spilsbury in a decade when it seemed that private violence was setting the tone for the war smouldering in Europe. He had taken rooms in central London to be nearer his work, while the family remained at Marlborough Hill. He still did most of his own clerical administration, although Alan, his eldest son, helped with some of the routine tasks. Spilsbury was one of those individuals who, today, would be called a workaholic.

When the Second World War was declared, Spilsbury was in his early sixties and the already over-worked pathologist saw his younger colleagues disappear into the armed forces, leaving behind them an ever-increasing workload. In May 1940, he suffered a minor stroke which proved to be a harbinger of tragedy to come. Typically, although convalescing, he insisted on appearing in court to give evidence at the trial of Udham Singh, a Sikh who shot dead Sir Michael O'Dwyer, a former Governor of the Punjab, at a public meeting in London. As he recovered his strength following the stroke and began to slip back into the familiar work routine, the Luftwaffe began its daylight bombing raids on London. This onslaught was to have tragic consequences for many families, including the Spilsburys, whose son, Peter, a house surgeon working at St Thomas's Hospital, was killed by a bomb which hit the out-patients department where he was working.

The effect of the loss of his son was put poignantly by Spilsbury's biographers: '. . . he was a changed man. It is agreed by all who knew him that he never recovered from the shock of Peter's death . . . from that day . . . he began to fail.' Like many who are stricken by grief, Spilsbury sought solace by devoting himself to his work. Yet the fates had more sorrow in store for him with the death in 1941 of his sister, Constance, with whom he had stayed at Hampstead after he was bombed out of his apartment in central London. And, then, in 1945, came the cruel loss of his son Alan from consumption.

Spilsbury had made his own singular contribution to the war in 1943 when his expert advice was sought by the planners of the deception which became known as *The Man Who Never Was*. This was the fabled exercise in which a corpse purporting to be that of a British Army Major carrying documents designed to mislead the Germans over Allied invasion plans, was launched from a submarine off the coast of Spain. The corpse selected for the role of dupe was that of a thirty-four-year-old vagrant who had died of neglect and pneumonia.

There was water in the man's lungs but it was not salt water as would have been the case in a person who drowned in the sea, which is what the Germans were expected to believe. With characteristic forthrightness, Spilsbury told the Allied planners not to worry because, to spot the discrepancy 'would need a pathologist of my experience, and there aren't any in Spain.' What might have been a risky strategy turned out brilliantly and the Germans were deceived into believing the Allies would invade Greece when in fact they landed in Sicily. As the world rejoiced at the cessation of global conflict, Spilsbury's life lay in ruins, shattered by domestic tragedy.

For six years, since 1941, he had lived in a small hotel at Frognal in north London. The young man who had taken long, solitary walks as an undergraduate, lived a lonely life during his twilight years. He came down to breakfast but was rarely seen at other mealtimes. He divided his time between London's mortuaries and coroners' courts and the laboratory at University College in Gower Street, where he often worked late at night. He saw his daughter regularly and, when he was not working, spent weekends with his family and friends.

This was a bearable life during the extraordinary days of the war years, but after he suffered the loss of his two sons, he began to collapse inwardly and to think of his own frailties. At the age of sixty-eight, arthritic and slightly stooping, he looked older than his years, and a lifetime of self-imposed toil started to take its toll. Friends and colleagues noticed how the man with the once sure technique began to fumble and work with hands that had lost their fluent skills. Superintendent Robert Fabian, better known as 'Fabian of the Yard', who knew Spilsbury well, commented on the pathologist's decline after the post-mortem examination he carried out on Alec de Antiquis.

This tragic case, in which de Antiquis, an heroic member of the public, was shot dead by armed raiders in a London street following a robbery at a jewellery shop in April 1947, proved to be a watershed in the criminal use of firearms. It also turned out to be Spilsbury's last big case. He seemed perplexed when he could not find an exit wound for the bullet which had been fired into the victim's head. It was Fabian who solved the puzzle by picking up the bullet which had lodged in the entry wound and fallen out during examination. Whatever effect this may have had on those present, there can be little doubt that it further undermined Spilsbury's own sense of diminishing confidence in his abilities.

Sir Bentley Purchase, one of Spilsbury's closest associates for many years, had observed his friend's failing powers during the previous year when he had inadvertently submitted two separate reports for the same post-mortem examination. For a meticulous man like Spilsbury who had denied himself the support of secretarial assistance all his working life, preferring to rely on his own resources and power of memory, this must have further dented his pride. Purchase and other coroners did their best as loyal colleagues to give him cases in central London in order to minimise his need to travel and the fatigue that went with it. He suffered from insomnia and, it is thought, he had another stroke while alone in his hotel room. His arthritis grew worse and he was prone to bronchitis – he was a man coming to the end of his tether, both physically and mentally.

The signs that he was preparing to end it all were present but acquired significance only in retrospect. It had long been Spilsbury's practice to order his post-mortem forms in batches of 500. In 1947, he put in an order for only 200. As he used them up, they became like leaves falling from his tree of life. He was down to a mere handful of forms when he decided to terminate his life. He had already written to his friend, Dr Eric Gardner, who was on holiday in Switzerland, telling him that by the time he received the letter, 'it would be all over'.

The day he chose was 17 December 1947. It began with the scrupulously observed routine of a man of habit. He breakfasted at his hotel and went to the garage at Hampstead to pick up his car. He drove first to St Pancras coroner's court and then back to Hampstead, where he carried out his last post-mortem on a woman who had died while undergoing a surgical operation. In the afternoon, he returned his car to the garage at Hampstead, gave the staff Christmas tips and told them he would not need the car again before the holiday.

When he went back to his hotel, he had to ring the bell to gain entry, for he had left his front door key lying on the dressing table in his room. He explained that he had forgotten something. Then he went to his laboratory at University College in Gower Street where he destroyed various papers and documents. He also used his last post-mortem form to record his findings in the examination he had made earlier in the day. Uncharacteristically, he sealed it in an envelope with an explanatory note, addressed to Sir Bentley Purchase, and posted it himself. After dining early at his club where he handed the hall porter the key to his private locker, saying he would no longer be needing it, he returned to the Gower Street laboratory at 7.30 p.m.

At about 8.10 p.m., a technician at the hospital returning to his workbench noticed a light on in Spilsbury's room and smelled gas. He knocked, and when he received no reply, tried the door which was locked. He called a watchman who opened the door with a pass key. They found Spilsbury lying on the floor. He was still alive and artificial respiration was attempted. By the time that Purchase arrived, following an urgent summons, efforts at revival had failed and his friend expired within the shadow of the filing cabinets containing his records of thousands of cases.

Sir Bentley Purchase presided over the inquest, a sad affair at which most of the participants were friends or professional associates of the dead man. Police Constable Shreeve, the coroner's officer at St Pancras, who had known Spilsbury for twenty-five years, had observed his declining powers in the post-mortem room. And Mrs Evelyn Steel, his daughter, who had seen her father regularly right up to the end, said he had spoken of being tired. Dr R.H.D. Short, pathologist at University College Hospital, found that Spilsbury had died of coronary thrombosis and carbon monoxide poisoning.

Purchase asked if Spilsbury's heart ailment was necessarily a fatal condition. Dr Short believed that it would eventually have resulted in death. He added, 'It is quite certain that a person of Sir Bernard's knowledge and attainments would be bound to realise its dangerous condition himself.' There was no suicide note, other than the intimation given in his letter to Dr Gardner, but his every action on the final day of his life was that of a person tidying up in preparation for the end. Purchase could give but one verdict which was that Spilsbury had taken his own life. Holding back his grief, the coroner added, 'I am quite sure this was not the Sir Bernard who had made such a reputation. His mind was not as it used to be.'

In the years that have elapsed since Sir Bernard Spilsbury's death, it has become fashionable to criticise him. He was a shy and modest man and, if he was regarded as infallible, it was not because he claimed to be. Others, impressed by his authority, thrust infallibility upon him. It is true that his confidence, combined with a natural authority, gave rise to suggestions of arrogance. If he had ever written the book he planned on forensic medicine, he might have analysed the presentation of expert evidence. He might have discussed the balance of doubts and certainties that are the grounds of decision-making and which, no doubt, he always considered in his own cases. He did his agonising in private – that was in keeping with his temperament as a loner. But, when called to give account in court, he swerved not nor vacillated an instant. His opinions were clear and succinctly put, expressing his honestly held interpretation of the evidence at the time. If he was wrong, if his technique was at fault, it was up to others to show cause. Indeed, his opponents did try and frequently failed, witness the various confrontations with Robert Bronte.

The *British Medical Journal* mourned the passing of 'one of the most distinguished figures in forensic medicine'. Spilsbury was certainly that, and despite his shortcomings, fallibility being one of them, his greatness lay in the new confidence which he injected into forensic pathology. The subject had lain somewhat neglected when he came to the scene at the beginning of the twentieth century, and, in the course of forty years, he raised it to an unprecedented level of public awareness. Forensic science acquired a new status in the medico-legal framework and the role of the expert had been revitalised.

Although he had been the subject of professional jealousy, especially over the incident which precipitated his departure from St Mary's, Spilsbury, because he was a loner and because he quickly achieved status, did not indulge in the petty behaviour which otherwise tended to mar a great profession. But in the years after his death, when his work was judged by others and his contribution assessed, strong criticism was voiced of his conduct and standing.

Sir Sydney Smith, who had endured a number of encounters with Spilsbury, wrote of his fellow pathologist that, 'His belief in himself was so strong that he could not conceive the possibility of error either in his observation or interpretation.' He acknowledged him as a 'man of outstanding brilliance and complete integrity' who was 'so often right that he could be forgiven for being stubborn when he was wrong'. Having said that, he mourned him sincerely. Smith added, 'One might almost hope that there will never be another Bernard Spilsbury.'

Of course, there never will be, although there have been those who have aspired to his mantle. The bone of contention that his inheritors had with him was that he would not change his mind in face of what they regarded in particular instances as superior logic. As Sydney Smith put it, 'Once he had committed himself to an opinion he would never change it.' Once the oracle had spoken, that was that. J.D. Cassels QC, who unsuccessfully defended Sidney Fox, called this 'an unhealthy state' and complained at the trial that 'it will be a sorry day for the administration of justice in this land if we are to be thrust into such a position that, because Sir Bernard Spilsbury expressed an opinion, it is of such weight that it is impossible to question it.'

The fact is that his opinions were challenged all the time, on occasions against almost overwhelming odds, as in the Thorne case, where he was confronted in court by six doctors who argued against him. That his opinions won the day may mean no more than that they were the most convincing. Like many powerful men, he probably was unaware of the strength of his own influence but he was certainly not lacking in conviction. Sneaking admiration for his style came through in Sydney Smith's remark that, together with Willcox and Roche Lynch, Spilsbury 'set a high standard for all future medical experts to aim at.'

Keith Simpson was less charitable in his remarks about Spilsbury whom he described as a 'monolith, alone, aloof, respected but unloved: and unmourned too, when he finally committed suicide, in his tiny laboratory in University College, London.' Simpson faulted the man for not working or lecturing abroad, for not attending international congresses, not consulting with such contemporaries as Smith or Glaister, for not writing a textbook or contributing to the literature of his subject and for not encouraging students to work with him. It is an impressive list of failures to include in the epitaph of a man whose name was a household word, yet the observations, in essence, are correct. Spilsbury was remarkable in his single-mindedness and his belief in his own powers which was why, in the end, when he saw his strength ebbing away, he took his own life.

The private man with the lone instinct was made famous and turned into a public figure by popular acclaim after the Crippen trial. It was probably his elevation to the status of a public figure which so irked some of Spilsbury's contemporaries and later detractors. But, in the 1920s and '30s, the public wanted to indulge its courtroom heroes such as Curtis Bennett, Marshall Hall and others, because they added drama and character to otherwise sombre judicial proceedings.

Newspaper reporting of the great criminal trials was at its peak and, while most of those who stood accused of murder were portrayed as evil midgets, those who defended and prosecuted them were giants. Spilsbury, erect of stance, firm of jaw and sure of speech, was cast in a giant mould and 'the coming man' satisfied public demand. He made no claims to greatness or infallibility for himself and it was not in his nature to dwell on his reputation. His desire was to pursue his chosen craft for the public benefit without equivocation and to the very best of his ability. He was a man for his time, no more and no less.

Chapter Two

THE PATRIARCH

Sir Sydney Smith

EGYPT IN THE 1920s was a place of political ferment. The British Government had ended its protectorate status in 1922 and announced that the country was an independent sovereign state with its own king. In practice, the British High Commissioner counselled the sovereign and every government minister had a British adviser. The country remained under martial law, which had been in force since 1914 against a background of civil unrest.

In January 1924, Said Pasha Zaghloul, the nationalist leader who had been exiled by the British, returned to the country and was elected Prime Minister. He beat a path to London for talks with the British Government about full independence but returned to Egypt empty-handed when the talks broke down. The atmosphere in Cairo was tense and the flashpoint came on 19 November 1924.

Soon after midday, Sir Lee Stack Pasha, the Sirdar, or Commander-in-Chief, of the Egyptian Army and Governor-General of the Sudan, left his office at the War Ministry to return home. He was driven through the busy streets of Cairo accompanied by his aide-de-camp, Captain Patrick Campbell. As the driver slowed the car to negotiate the traffic in the centre of the city, several gunmen appeared at the roadside and fired a number of shots at the occupants of the car.

Although wounded, the Sirdar's driver accelerated to put his car beyond reach of the gunmen, and drove to the British Residency. Lord Allenby, Special High Commissioner for Egypt, was taking lunch with Herbert Asquith when their meal was interrupted by the news of the assassination attempt. Sir Lee Stack, mortally wounded, was carried into the drawing room and help was summoned. The Sirdar had been hit with several shots and he died the following day in the Anglo-American Hospital. The gunmen had made a clean getaway in a waiting car.

News of the assassination caused anger and consternation in London. The popular view was that the killing had been masterminded by Zaghloul and there were anxieties at the consequences for Egyptian claims for independence. In the middle of the crisis involving soldiers and diplomats there emerged the unlikely figure of Dr Sydney Smith. Since 1917 he had been in charge of the medico-legal section at the Parquet, a department of the Egyptian Ministry of Justice responsible for the investigation of crime.

Smith was well versed in the examination of firearms evidence, for his time in Egypt had coincided with the country's period of unrest and there had been ample opportunity to study crimes of violence. He probably did not realise it at the time but he was about to become a pioneer in the field of forensic ballistics. A reconstruction of the crime was ordered and an examination made of all the spent cartridge cases found at the scene of the shooting and of the bullets retrieved from the victim's bodies.

The nine cartridge cases were all of .32 automatic pistol ammunition and the marks on them indicated that they had been fired from three different weapons identified as a Mauser, a Browning and a Colt. Five of the bullets, including the one which had killed Sir Lee Stack, had been modified as dumdum ammunition by cutting a cross into their metal tips. The fatal bullet bore marks characteristic of having been fired from a Colt pistol with a well worn-barrel.

Because of the prevalence in Egypt of crimes committed with firearms, Dr Sydney Smith had adopted an experimental technique being developed in the USA. This involved combining the optical systems of two microscopes in order to compare two different specimens side-by-side in the same field of vision. Thus it became possible to examine and compare bullets and cartridge cases in minute detail.

When Smith examined the bullet which had killed the Sirdar, he saw a familiar mark on it. Between the normal rifling grooves scratched on the bullet as it spiralled its way out of the gun's barrel was another wider groove which he had seen before. The bullet had been fired from a weapon with a defect in its muzzle which left its characteristic mark. What was significant about it was that he had seen exactly that same mark on bullets recovered from a number of previous murders. With characteristic boldness, he told the officers in charge of the investigation that he could identify the murder weapon.

Making full use of informers and acting on 'information received', police officers hunting the Sirdar's assassins narrowed their search to a group of nationalists led by Shafik Mansour, a lawyer who had been arrested several times on suspicion of murder. Initial enquiries failed to produce any useful evidence so the police decided to use a spy. Two of the assassins were quickly identified as the Ennayat brothers whom it was thought would confess if they realised the inevitability of being convicted.

A ruse was devised based on Smith's belief that if he could lay his hands on the brothers' guns, he would be able to confirm them as the murder weapons. The brothers were therefore advised by the spy to make a run for it in the expectation that they would take their weapons with them. They reacted as expected and fell neatly into the trap laid for them. They were arrested on a train which they believed would carry them beyond the reach of the authorities. A basket of fruit in their possession was searched and four automatic pistols and a quantity of ammunition were found.

Two of the weapons were .25 calibre pistols and hence of no immediate interest to the murder investigation. But the remaining guns were both .32 calibre, one a Browning or Sûreté type and the other, a Colt. Smith took the two .32 pistols to his laboratory and in a tense atmosphere with the Chief of Police and Director of Public Security looking on, test-fired them into boxes containing cotton wool. This was a standard procedure to ensure that the only marks made on the bullets would be those left by the guns.

The test bullets and cartridge cases were put under the comparison microscope and viewed next to the bullets and casings taken from the scene of the Sirdar's assassination. The results showed that the Sûreté pistol had been fired three times at the murder scene and the Colt was clearly identified as the murder weapon on account of the flaw in its barrel which left the characteristic mark on bullets if fired. With some excitement, Sydney Smith wrote later, 'I was able to say with absolute certainty that this pistol, and no other, had fired the bullet that killed the Sirdar.'

Faced with the certainty of conviction, the Ennayat brothers confessed and implicated others in the assassination incident. In the mopping-up operation which followed, police arrested six others, including the gang leader, Shafik Mansour, and located the workshop containing the tools used to convert the bullets into 'dum-dum' ammunition.

The trial of the eight men accused of conspiring to kill Sir Lee Stack was held in May 1925. Dr Sydney Smith gave evidence for the prosecution. Asked if any of the pistols featuring as exhibits had been used in the shooting, he picked up the Colt and held it above his head; in his other hand, he held a jeweller's lens. Referring to the defect in its barrel which left a tell-tale mark on bullets fired from it, he said, 'I declare definitely that they (the murder bullets) were both fired from this Colt.' The eight assassins were found guilty and sentenced to death. Seven were hanged and one had his sentence commuted to life imprisonment.

The outcome was a triumph for Smith and his application of a little-known scientific procedure. The doctor with his jeweller's lens became a much-admired figure and, like Sir Bernard Spilsbury, made a signal contribution to the development of forensic medicine. Smith was a pragmatist. When his former tutor, Professor Harvey Littlejohn, visited him in Cairo, a batch of Marsh Test apparatus sets for identifying arsenic became a subject for discussion. 'Why do you need so many?' asked Littlejohn. 'Homicides,' replied Smith with disarming simplicity. He applied the same criterion to the need to cope with crimes involving fire-arms – find a technique that works and use it.

The contrast between Sydney Smith's birthplace in New Zealand and that of Spilsbury in England could hardly have been greater. The distance separating Roxburgh, Otago from Leamington, Warwickshire is considerable but the social and environmental gulf in the last century was enormous. Smith's father was a road builder in an underdeveloped region inhabited by goldminers and sheep farmers, whereas Spilsbury senior was a professional man in a prosperous town. Despite the differences, there was one common thread – both families had a love of learning and culture.

Smith was born in Roxburgh in August 1883 and, as a schoolboy, came under the spell of a perceptive village schoolmaster. Stimulated at school and encour-aged by his parents, young Smith decided he wanted to see the world and believed that the best way of achieving his ambition was to become a doctor.

He began his scientific education in unfashionable Roxburgh by working as apprentice to the local pharmacist. This provided a useful stepping stone to the position of chemist's assistant in Dunedin and opened the door to formal tuition and the chance to gain some qualifications. At the age of twenty-three, Smith qualified as a pharmacist and started to earn a modest salary. He at once began to study for entrance to the University of New Zealand and, in due course, enrolled as a part-time student at Victoria College, Wellington.

He combined his studies with his job of dispensing pharmacist at Wellington Hospital and thus could claim a toe-hold in the world of medicine. The aspir-ing doctor achieved good results and in 1908 he decided that Edinburgh was the place to learn his chosen profession. Using money saved from his earnings as a pharmacist, he made the first of many long journeys from the Antipodes to Scotland. There he secured a scholarship worth £100 for three years and settled down to study at one of the world's great centres of medical learning. He cher-ished his early experiences of Edinburgh and, years later, the student was destined to return as master.

Sydney Smith qualified as a newly fledged medical practitioner in 1912. He gained a first class degree and also won a research scholarship. The young man about to make his mark on the world thought it prudent to share his life and he married soon after graduating. Kitty would be his 'good companion for half a century' as he described her in his memoirs.

He embarked on a career in forensic medicine almost by accident. He worked in general practice for a month as a *locum tenens* in Fife, but concluded from the experience that he was not cut out to be a GP. Ophthalmology was the subject he chose for his research scholarship and he had just started at the Eye Department of Edinburgh's Royal Infirmary when he was interviewed by the Dean of the Faculty, Professor Harvey Littlejohn.

Littlejohn was also Professor of Forensic Medicine in the university and had succeeded his father Henry in the Chair. He was part of the rich Scottish tradition of forensic medicine, being to Edinburgh what the Glaisters, father and son, were to Glasgow. Littlejohn saw potential in the young New Zealander and talked him into becoming an assistant in his department at a salary of £50 a year. Thus began Sydney Smith's journey into forensic medicine, a branch of learning that Scotland had put on the map in 1807 by establishing the first professional Chair of its kind in the English-speaking world.

Edinburgh is the true home of the forensic arts in Britain, for, in addition to the city's pioneering lead in the teaching of forensic medicine, it was also the spiritual home of Sherlock Holmes. The great fictional detective, famed for his investigative genius, was the creation of Sir Arthur Conan Doyle who, as a young man, had studied medicine at Edinburgh Royal Infirmary. One of his tutors was a distinguished surgeon, Joseph Bell, a doctor with an enviable reputation for his diagnostic skills. He was also renowned for his powers of observation which he used to study his patients' appearance and thereby deduce the nature of their occupation and character.

Bell urged his students to use all their faculties before coming to a decision about anything. It was admirable advice for a young man in any profession but for a doctor it was particularly significant. Merely by observing one of his patients and without questioning or examining him, Bell informed a group of students that the man was left-handed and a shoe-repairer by trade. Explaining himself to both patient and students, Bell remarked that the worn patches on the trousers were caused by gripping a lap stone between the knees and the fact that the right side was more worn than the other indicated that the cobbler wielded the hammer in his left hand. Conan Doyle recognised this perceptive gift and moulded it into the character of Sherlock Holmes with the telling force that emerged with his stories.

The spirit of Joseph Bell permeated the lecture theatres at Edinburgh and by the time Sydney Smith studied there, Sherlock Holmes was well established in the nation's reading habits. Smith soon concluded that his chosen field of specialisation required more than observation and deduction – knowledge had to be acquired and experience gained. After all, forensic medicine, or medical jurisprudence as it was more formally called, was an amalgam of two great professions – medicine and law. In some instances, the association with law enforcement was very close and at Edinburgh, Harvey Littlejohn, in addition to being the University's Professor of Forensic Medicine, was also Chief Surgeon to the City Police. Moreover, some aspects of the forensic pathologist's job were hardly medical, such as the examination of firearms, cartridge cases and bullets, a field in which Sydney Smith was to gain pre-eminence. This work was directed to the pathologist on account of his knowledge of gunshot wounds; also, because in an age before forensic science became established in its own right, the doctors were the custodians of such scientific knowledge that could be applied to the investigation of crime.

After a short spell understudying the master, Smith was given his first major investigation. In June 1913, two ploughmen came across a mysterious object float-ing in a water-filled quarry near Winchburgh in West Lothian. Their first reaction was that a passing vandal had thrown a farmer's scarecrow into the quarry where it lay waterlogged and spread-eagled to frighten passers-by. On closer inspection, the two men realised that the object was not one but two human shapes tied together with window cord. With the aid of a tree branch, they dragged out what proved to be the bodies of two fully clothed, long dead children.

The local police had received no reports of any missing children and there was no information on which to start an investigation. Indeed the doctor called to the scene believed that a post-mortem examination of the corpses would be a waste of time in view of the state of decomposition which was so advanced as to have rendered their features unrecognisable. The pathologist took the view that this made it even more necessary to carry out an autopsy in the hope of provid-ing the police with some information whereby the youngsters could be traced.

Smith began by examining the remnants of rotten clothing clinging to the bodies. The children were dressed alike and on one of the shirts he observed a laundry mark which proved to be the imprint of a poorhouse at Dysart in Fife. The clothing yielded no further clues, so attention was directed to the bodies, which exhibited the phenomenon known as adipocere whereby their fat had been converted to a firm, wax-like consistency. This is an unusual condition which occurs over a long period when a body is subjected to damp conditions such as immersion in water or burial in damp ground. The process is one in which the neutral body fats are hydrolysed into a mixture of fatty acids and soap with the result that the body, especially the limbs, retain much of their original shape.

In the remains which confronted Sydney Smith, the bodies had been wholly transformed into adipocere, with the exception of their feet. As his examina-tion progressed, the pathologist was able to establish that both victims were male and, from measurements of their height, he determined that one was aged about six to seven years and the other about four. These estimates were confirmed by examining the teeth which, in the case of the elder boy, showed that his first permanent molars had come through; this tended to confirm his age as about six years. The younger boy had all his milk teeth and as none of his permanent teeth had emerged, his age was put at between two and four years. Inspection of the epiphyses, the soft growing ends of the long bones, in the elder boy confirmed an age of around six or seven years.

Examination of the internal organs showed them to be normal, although remarkably well preserved. Of particular interest was the content of the stomachs which had also been preserved intact. In both bodies, the stomachs contained a quantity of material which included easily identified vegetables; peas, barley, potatoes, turnips and leeks. All the ingredients, as Smith readily recognised, of nourishing Scotch broth. This material which had been preserved by the adipocerous covering of the bodies was of particular importance in helping to establish time of death. The partially digested nature of the stomach contents suggested that the boys had eaten their last meal about one hour before they died. The disused quarry where the boys were found was in a secluded area reached by a long, winding cart track. The likelihood was that the two youngsters had fallen foul of someone with local knowledge, probably a person known to them; possibly even a parent.

The pathologist's medical detective work had thus provided a few facts for the police to build up an investigation. The adipocerous state of the bodies suggested death had occurred between eighteen months and two years previously, and hence the boys would have gone missing during the late summer or autumn of 1911. Their ages were known fairly precisely and also their heights. The shabby quality of their clothing combined with the poorhouse stamp on one of the shirts indicated impoverished family circumstances. Armed with these details the police soon discovered that two boys, aged seven and four years, had disappeared from the Winchburgh area in November 1911. Their father, Patrick Higgins, a former soldier, was a widower who had been imprisoned for failing to maintain his children. The two boys were looked after in the poorhouse at Dysart while their father served his jail sentence.

Enquiries among local men who knew Higgins made it plain that he had been seen with the boys one night in November and, when asked how they were, replied that he had found a home for them. The police swiftly collected a number of witnesses' statements which justified issuing a warrant for Higgins's arrest. He was apprehended in Broxburn and, in due course, tried for murder at the High Court of Justiciary in Edinburgh. His defence, based on a history of epilepsy, was that he was of unsound mind when he killed his sons. Despite medical evidence supporting this claim, the jury brought in a guilty verdict by unanimous decision but with a recommendation to mercy on account of the time which had elapsed since the crime was committed.

Higgins was not granted a reprieve and his execution was fixed for 1 October 1913. Sydney Smith attended the hanging. 'It was the first time I had seen a man hanged,' he wrote in his autobiography, 'and I found it rather an unpleasant experience; especially as I had been partly instrumental in bringing him to the gallows.' Smith also gave a dispassionate account of the execution, remarking that the magistrates' clerk had assured news reporters afterwards that Higgins had been calm and his death instantaneous. It worried Smith that when he tested the pulse of the executed man, a feeble heartbeat was still discernible. He accepted that with the neck broken and the spinal cord severed, death was practically instantaneous. But there was always the nagging doubt that, with continued circulation of the blood, a degree of consciousness might still be present.

Alongside Smith's evident compassion went his hard-headedness. He had the teacher's instincts and as his first important case had presented him with an uncommon example of adipocere, he resolved to keep a specimen for subsequent demonstration purposes. With Harvey Littlejohn's startled approval he secured his specimens – two heads, an assortment of limbs and the internal organs – which he had parcelled up and took with him on the train to Edinburgh. He and Littlejohn survived a nervous journey, ignoring the quizzical looks from fellow passengers disturbed by the unpleasant stench which seemed to be associated with their luggage. The specimens of adipocere ended up in the University's Forensic Medicine Museum where they were used to teach generations of students.

Thoroughly captivated by his first encounter in the realm of forensic medicine, Sydney Smith decided to drop his part-time ophthalmology work and to take up public health which was a better complementary discipline. By 1914, he had obtained an MD and taken a Diploma in Public Health which qualified him to move up the career ladder. In the summer of that year, he applied for the position of assistant to Dr Hamilton, Principal Medico-Legal Expert to the Egyptian Government. He was accepted for the post but the wheels of bureaucracy in Cairo ground so slowly that, tired of waiting, he took a job in his native New Zealand.

Smith was on board a ship bound for New Zealand when events in Europe led to the outbreak of the First World War. On reaching his destination he took up his position as Medical Officer of Health for Otago based at Dunedin but volunteered at once for military service. His application was not immediately accepted but in due course he joined the New Zealand Army Corps and carried out medical duties at various military camps which paralleled his civilian public health work. Despite a number of ingenious attempts to join the momentous events taking place on the other side of the world, he stayed in New Zealand until 1917, when he was summoned to Egypt.

Dr Hamilton had died unexpectedly and the government in Cairo cabled Dr Smith offering him the post of Principal Medico-Legal Expert which carried with it a lectureship in forensic medicine. The New Zealand Government raised no objection and the itinerant pathologist sailed for Egypt on board a troopship carrying men to the Middle East.

The medico-legal department which he inherited from Dr Hamilton was attached to the Ministry of Justice, known, rather curiously, as the Parquet, a French word referring to the floor of the courtroom. Egyptian law was not based on the British system but followed the Napoleonic Code. The head of the Parquet was the Procurator-General who controlled the police and decided which criminal cases should be sent for trial. His officers were magistrates who had powers to examine witnesses and make decisions about prosecutions.

The medico-legal section was part of this system and its employees were government officials. The late Dr Hamilton had pioneered the use of medical science in the investigation of crime in Egypt in the early days of such novelties as X-ray examination. In 1904, the distinguished Egyptologists, Mr (later Sir) Elliot Smith and Howard Carter, had caused a stir in Cairo by riding in a taxicab, with the mummy of Tuthmosis VI as a passenger, on their way to an X-ray unit. The section was not as comprehensively equipped as the new incumbent would have liked and he particularly regretted the lack of laboratory facilities. Such scientific analyses as the section required were carried out at either the School of Medicine or the Government Laboratory. Arthur Lucas, Director of the Chemical Department at the Government Laboratory was a distinguished forensic chemist and an enthusiastic collaborator. Nevertheless, Smith wanted to be able to carry out his own analytical work and he made the establishment of a laboratory one of his first priorities.

There followed an exciting period for the young pathologist, building up one of the finest medico-legal departments in the world and investigating a rich variety of cases. The Land of the Pharaohs with its fascinating history and singular customs was also a violent society which experienced a high murder rate. Smith viewed this as something of an anomaly, for he found the Egyptians to be good-natured and gentle people on the whole. Nevertheless, his services were called on to investigate 1,000 murder cases in one year. Indeed, as he put it many years later in his memoirs, 'Murder was a business'.

This was amply borne out by a mass murder which came to light in Alexandria in 1920. Workmen excavating a trench stumbled across a mass grave as the result of unearthing some human bones when the side of the trench collapsed and undermined the floor of an adjacent house. Under Smith's supervision, the earthen floor of the house was carefully taken up and the full extent of the discovery was exposed. Fourteen bodies, buried in two layers, were found in varying states of decomposition. All had been strangled and some of the corpses still had the ligatures fastened around their necks. Post-mortem examination confirmed that the victims were exclusively adult females, but it was Smith's new-found understanding of Moslem customs which gave him a clue as to their origins. The women had all been circumcised which confirmed they were Moslems and yet, unusually, they still had their pubic hair. For reasons of hygiene it was the practice for women to shave that part of their body; the exceptions to this habit were prostitutes who believed their pubic hair had aphrodisiac properties.

Like prostitutes everywhere, the ladies of the street in Alexandria were vulnerable to violent predators and frequently disappeared as a result. With the help of the police, Smith was able to identify most of the dead women who had gone missing over a period of about two years. Understandably, the owners of the house with the mass grave under its floors were being urgently sought after. Two couples were eventually arrested and their sordid murder-for-profit scheme was revealed.

One of the characteristics of Egyptian prostitutes was that they carried their wealth about with them in the form of jewellery. They had no use for banks and converted their earnings to gold and jewellery which they wore as ornaments. Unfortunately, there were those who could see that apart from the normal dangers of their calling they also represented tempting targets for robbery. The foursome in the house in Alexandria contrived a system whereby the women patrolled the streets looking for suitably bejewelled prostitutes who they lured back to the house for the ostensible purpose of selling their services to a rich landowner. Once inside the house, they were easy prey for one of the men who slipped a noose over their heads and throttled them. The murder victim was then stripped of her finery and precious ornaments and her corpse buried under the floor. The perpetrators of these crimes were brought to justice and suffered the death penalty.

In part, the prevailing tide of violence stemmed from the social structure of the country in which men were allowed to take four wives. Polygamy, despite its seeming attractions to the Western mind, was a source of strife, stimulating jealousy and bitter emotions over disputed inheritances. Under Moslem law, divorce was possible without the legal formalities customary in other places. It was possible, therefore, for a man to have a succession of wives, taking on a new partner when he tired of the current one. There was a snag though, for a wife despatched and effectively divorced in an ill-considered moment could not readily be taken back if her original husband changed his mind. She had first to be married and divorced from another man, a provision which was exploited by entrepreneurial marriage brokers. Bribery and all kinds of chicanery were used to settle disputes and, when all else failed, there was always murder.

One of the problems resulting from these social practices arose over the maintenance of the children. A divorced woman had custody of boys until the age of seven and girls up to the age of nine years, with her former husband bound by law to provide maintenance. A much-married and frequently divorced man was likely to carry a heavy financial burden providing for his offspring. The system also created problems over inheritance and a wife might attempt to eliminate the children of a rival in order to construct a situation in which her own children would inherit.

One outcome of this social order was a high rate of murder for elimination, and children were frequently the victims. Poisoning with arsenic to relieve the burden of maintenance or to carve the way to an inheritance was commonplace. It was an occurrence which kept Sydney Smith's laboratory busy and he noted the surprise on Harvey Littlejohn's face when, on a visit to Cairo, he noticed the dozen or so arsenic test kits standing on the bench. The Marsh Test, developed by an English chemist in 1836, was the standard procedure for detecting arsenic in human tissues and body fluids. Smith told his startled teacher that arsenical poisoning was so prevalent in Egypt that rarely a day went by when he was not testing for the poison in a suspected murder case.

One of the nastier duties that falls to the forensic pathologist is to preside over the exhumation of corpses. In Egypt, where the climate necessitated quick burial, suspicions about the circumstances of a particular death might not reach official ears until well after the victim had been interred. Hence, exhumations were quite frequent. Fortunately, the manner of burial prevented the worst aspects of disinterment such as the stench and corruption of flesh commonplace in more temperate climes. The Egyptians neither enclosed their dead in coffins nor really buried them. The practice was to wrap the body in a shroud and put it either in a shallow grave or on the surface of the ground and cover it with stones.

Putrefaction within such a makeshift tomb occurred rapidly in the hot climate where the temperatures in the shade might vary between 90° to 100°F. Air flowed freely between the stones along with flies which infested the body within twenty-four hours. It was possible in these conditions for a body to disintegrate completely within four to eight weeks leaving nothing more than a collection of bones.

The problem for the pathologist was often one of identifying the victim of secret homicide from the fragments of the human form that survived the rapid process of disintegration after death. Smith quickly became an expert on the identification of skeletal remains. Egypt was a cosmopolitan society in which the Egyptian, Arab, African and European races lived and worked side-by-side. Homicide being no respecter of persons, it was thus important to establish racial origin as part of the identification of any set of human remains.

There are no definitive physical characteristics of a human skull or the bones of the skeleton by which racial origin may be determined. But there are telltale signs which the experienced practitioner can take into account along with other evidence. Observable differences in life, such as the strong prognathous face of the African or the long, narrow face and high brow of the Arab, may be discerned in differences of measurement between their skulls. Similar differences in the long bones of the arms and legs can be compared using a comparative index of measurement similar to the formulae used for calculating stature from individual bones.

Where an exhumed corpse had not been reduced to just a skeleton, the pathologist had more scope for his role as medical detective. This was a task for which Sydney Smith, with his Edinburgh training, was especially suited. The knowledge that a callus in the centre of the forehead marked a man as a devout Moslem, on account of his forehead constantly touching the ground in prayer, would no doubt have appealed to Dr Joseph Bell. Tattoo marks, scars and indications of occupation on the body and clothing all added to the information which aided the identification process.

The way in which patient examination of a few remains built up a complete story is illustrated by a case in which Smith's expertise was sought. An elderly, but healthy, Egyptian landowner had disappeared from his home and foul play was suspected. The rumour was that the old man had been murdered by his own son who had dismembered the body and buried it in a field. An informant told the police where to dig and human remains were duly discovered.

The pathologist was presented with a skull, some bone fragments, a quantity of decomposed tissue and some vestiges of clothing. By assessing the measurements of the skull, Smith determined that the remains were those of an Egyptian male and because all the bone sutures were closed, was able to put his age at over sixty years. All the teeth were gone, save three molars in the lower jaw, and the way in which they had worn indicated the man had been fitted with an upper denture. A piece of scalp still attached to the skull had embedded in it a few dark hairs which analysis showed had been dyed. What could be re-assembled of the long bones of the skeleton confirmed they were of an elderly man who, in life, had probably been about five feet nine inches tall. Pressure marks on the lower ends of the shin bones indicated that the man had been in the habit of squatting on his haunches, a characteristic that tended to confirm him as an Egyptian. Among the other material were the broken remains of the hyoid bone from the dead man's throat, the condition of which indicated death by strangulation.

Thus, Smith was able to identify the remains as those of an elderly Egyptian male, five feet nine inches tall, who dyed his hair and wore a denture in his upper jaw. This description matched exactly with that of the missing landowner and a search of his house turned up a denture plate which the pathologist was able to fit into the upper jaw. Of special relevance was the pattern of wear on the three remaining teeth in the lower jaw. This corresponded perfectly with the molars in the denture. Here was clinching evidence of identity but a final touch was the discovery of a pot of black hair dye that the old man had used to satisfy his vanity. Having established identity beyond doubt and confirmed that a murder had been committed, it was not long before the perpetrator was brought to justice. The landowner's son had killed his father and hoped that his dismemberment and disposal of the body would adequately conceal his crime. But he had reckoned without the persistence and skill of the forensic pathologist.

The extent and variety of domestic murder kept Sydney Smith and his colleagues busy but added to this was the violence resulting from political unrest. Egypt's quest for independence lay fairly dormant during the years of the First World War but, within days of the Armistice being signed in 1918, the claims were renewed. The nationalist leader, Said Pasha Zaghloul, had his request for independence turned down by the British Government, with the result that rioting broke out in Cairo and Alexandria. There was insurrection in the streets and Europeans were attacked. In one violent incident, eight British soldiers were taken off a train at Luxor and killed. The government responded by exiling Zaghloul and the other ringleaders to Malta. This had the effect of raising the temperature still further and the violence spread throughout the country.

The Smiths, in their flat in Cairo, were kept awake night after night by the sound of gunfire in the city. The pathologist was obliged to carry a handgun in case his life was threatened on his routine journeys to and from his office in the Parquet building. The mortuary was literally knee deep in bodies, most of them victims of gunshot wounds. Smith kept a supply of fifty large bottles of sulphuric acid in his first-floor laboratory as a weapon in the event that a mob attempted to take over. He kept on good terms with the Egyptians who perhaps recognised him as a colonial rather than an Englishman. Indeed he expressed his feelings of solidarity for local political aspirations when the First Secretary of the Residency asked him to join a group of senior officials to discuss the state of the country. Smith suggested that Egypt be granted Dominion status and that Zaghloul be allowed to return to his country, where he would undoubtedly be elected Prime Minister. 'Do have a whisky and soda before you go,' the First Secretary offered this purveyor of unfashionable views.

The 1918 riots were subdued but strong anti-British feelings smouldered on, regularly erupting into fresh bouts of violence. What the increasing use of firearms did for Sydney Smith was to provide him with first-hand professional experience of the damage caused by gunshot wounds. By extension, his post-mortem examination of such casualties led to his involvement in what he called 'the infant science of forensic ballistics'. It also led to further confrontations with officialdom.

Following the deaths of a number of people during a riot in Alexandria, the medico-legal department were asked to examine the wounds on the bodies with a view to identifying the weapons used against them. This necessitated exhuming the corpses of about fifty victims all of whom were supposed to have been killed by small arms fire discharged at them by rioters. What Smith and his colleagues discovered was that the wounds had been caused by .303 bullets fired by British troops. There was no doubt about the origin of the ammunition, for the lead core of the bullets was tipped with aluminium and encased in a cupro-nickel jacket. Only British ordnance factories made this type of ammunition and, as Smith reported to the War Office, it seemed that in some instances a paper pulp material had been substituted for the aluminium component of the bullets. It appeared that this was for reasons of economy and official assurances that the paper pulp was thoroughly sterilised in order not to create any wound infection was a concession to humanitarianism that he found somewhat ironic, given that bullets are intended to kill people.

Egypt was made an independent sovereign state in 1922, but both martial law and British authority remained intact. Every senior member of the Egyptian administration had a British adviser at his elbow and, so long as the British Army remained as an occupying force, real power still lay with London. There was a kind of uneasy truce for a while and, in July 1923, martial law was ended. The exiled Zaghloul was allowed to return and in January 1924 he was elected Prime Minister. It was the lull before the storm.

The murder of Sir Lee Stack in a dusty Cairo street precipitated a political furore and set back the course of Egyptian independence. While the police used their traditional methods of seeking leads to the crime from their network of informers, Sydney Smith was employing the latest scientific methods. He had turned his posting to a forensic backwater into a potential triumph by his insistence on building up a strong technical capability in his department. Alert to developments in other parts of the world, he read that the American firearms experts, Charles E. Waite and Philip O. Gravelle, had combined the optical systems of two microscopes in order to compare bullets. Smith experimented in his own laboratory and finished constructing his own comparison microscope a matter of weeks before Sir Lee Stack was shot dead.

Armed with his new technique, Smith was able to make an early breakthrough in the investigation of the murder, unequivocally identifying the murder weapons and thereby placing guilt on their owners. Some of the bullets fired during the incident had been hand-finished into dumdum projectiles. A search of the house of one of the suspects revealed tools including two engineer's vices which told their own story. Metallic dust particles clinging to the vices were shown to be identical to filings taken from the crime bullets. There was no clearer proof that the workshop in the house had been used to convert ordinary ammunition into the dumdum variety.

In his appreciation of Smith's contribution to forensic ballistics, crime historian, Jürgen Thorwald, wrote, 'At the end of May 1925, Sydney Smith stood up in court in what had come to be a characteristic pose, the murderer's Colt in one hand, his jeweller's lens in the other. He was testifying as the final witness for the prosecution. His findings were accepted without question, and sealed the fate of the conspirators.'

A brief reference to Smith's contribution was reported in the *British Medical Journal* in 1926 and, two years later, there was a full account by him in *The Police Journal*. In characteristic fashion, he referred to his use of the comparison microscopes as evolving 'slowly from a Heath Robinson affair'. Whatever its origins, Smith's use of the new method to aid a major murder investigation pre-dated the American Sacco and Vanzetti case by at least two years and Britain's Browne and Kennedy case by the same margin.

Despite the difficult times on Egypt's political front, Smith continued to teach at the School of Medicine at Kasr el Aine and, aided by his assistant Dr Ahmer Bey, he wrote his first book on forensic medicine which he intended should be printed in Arabic. There were no publishing outlets in Cairo in the mid-1920s so the redoubtable doctor decided to publish the book himself even to the extent of buying paper and supervising the block making. His determination was rewarded, for he had clearly seen a gap in the market and the book was a great success. This achievement was crowned for the authors by an invitation from King Fuad to attend an audience so that he might congratulate them. His Majesty was presented with a specially-bound copy of the textbook which he accepted for inclusion in the royal library.

For Sydney Smith this was the beginning of a distinguished literary thread in his career. In 1925, he published his *Forensic Medicine and Toxicology* which he modestly described as, 'probably the first really well-illustrated work on the subject in Great Britain'. The textbook included a comprehensive chapter on 'Wounds from Firearms', an area of specialisation in which he was undoubtedly an expert. This paved the way for his editorship of *Taylor's Principles and Practice of Medical Jurisprudence*, a work of great medical scholarship and learning, which in due course he would pass on to Keith Simpson, a forensic pathologist of the coming generation.

At the time of Smith's emergence as a leading figure on the forensic scene, Simpson was a student at Guy's in London. Another link in the chain of forensic evolution was being forged in Glasgow where John Glaister the younger was in general practice and researching his doctorate of science thesis on the subject of classifying mammalian hair. In due time, Glaister would succeed Smith in Egypt but, for the moment, 'The Patriarch' ruled supreme in his desert kingdom, building both his reputation and experience.

'On the whole, the desert is a pretty good place for murder,' Smith wrote in his memoirs. His reasons for saying this were, naturally, well-founded, for the desert is a quick destroyer of mortal flesh. Abandoned bodies are soon reduced to skeletons, thus making identification difficult. Apart from information regarding sex, race, age, height and build which could be gleaned from the bones of long dead human beings, Smith became adept at interpreting other phenomena. In one case there was an abnormal flexion in the hip joints of a skeleton, suggesting that at some stage the body had been doubled up. Remnants of rotted sacking at the scene led him to believe that the body had been thrust into a sack. Such proved to be the case when the murder suspect confessed to his crime. Bullets, bones, fingerprints, clothing and bloodstains were all part of the pathologist's stock-in-trade.

Whereas the details of Spilsbury's cases were faithfully recorded on his file cards but sadly never collated into a textbook, Smith used his case experience to very good effect. Editions of his *Forensic Medicine* published well into the 1940s, and still carried illustrations which derived from his work in Egypt.

One of the founding fathers of forensic science in Britain was Dr Alfred Swaine Taylor who, at the age of twenty-eight, was appointed Professor of Medical Jurisprudence at Guy's Hospital Medical School. The first edition of his influential textbook was published in 1836 and has been in print ever since. Like Smith in the next century, he had the opportunity to study the use of firearms and the wounds they inflicted at close hand. In his case it was in Paris during the 1830 revolution. Taylor's textbook was regarded as the 'bible' by students of forensic medicine and it was perhaps fitting that Sydney Smith should succeed to its editorship. The appointment was certainly a mark of the high esteem in which he was held.

While on leave in Edinburgh in the summer of 1926, Smith and his wife called on Harvey Littlejohn. He found his friend and mentor in a troubled state. On 5 April, Littlejohn had carried out a post-mortem examination on the body of fifty-year-old Mrs Bertha Merrett. She had died of a gunshot wound to the side of the head in a position usually consistent with suicide. The casualty doctor at the Royal Infirmary who examined Mrs Merrett when she was admitted saw none of the usual signs associated with a suicidal head wound. There was an absence of tearing around the wound entry and no evidence of any powder deposits or singeing commonly seen in close-range gunshot wounds.

Smith thought it looked like a case of murder and this contention was borne out by the results of tests carried out with the weapon involved. Littlejohn was convinced and wrote a second report stating his opinion that suicide and accident could be ruled out, leaving murder as the likely option. The dead woman's son, Donald, who had been in the house at the time of the shooting, was arrested and charged.

Donald Merrett was tried in February and it was in many ways a north-south confrontation of experts. The full weight of Scottish forensic expertise was assembled on behalf of the Crown from both Edinburgh and Glasgow – Harvey Littlejohn and John Glaister senior aided by Sydney Smith and Glaister junior. They were ranged against the mighty Spilsbury, backed by Robert Churchill, the gun expert, for the defence. The outcome, which is included in Chapter One, was a stalemate in the sense that the verdict of 'Not Proven' allowed Merrett his freedom after serving twelve months in prison for forgery. But, ultimately, the moral victory went to the Scots, for Smith's prophetic words at the time, 'That is not the last we'll hear of young Merrett,' were fulfilled many years later. In 1954, Merrett murdered his wife and mother-in-law and subsequently committed suicide.

The Merrett trial proved to be a turning point for Smith. He believed that the stress created by the case was a contributory factor to Harvey Littlejohn's death in 1927. When he visited his former teacher in hospital before returning to Egypt, Littlejohn extracted a promise from him that he would come back to take his place when he died. Smith diverted the conversation away from such morbid considerations but, ten days later, Littlejohn was dead. Shortly after his return to Cairo, Smith received a letter from the Dean of the Faculty of Medicine in Edinburgh inviting him to apply for the post of Professor of Forensic Medicine. The position is a Regius Chair, being made not by the university but by the Crown. A letter soon arrived from the Secretary of State for Scotland offering Smith the appointment of the most prestigious Chair of Forensic Medicine in Britain.

After much heart-searching but with their young children's education at the forefront of their minds, the Smiths decided to return to Britain. Sydney had spent eleven years in Egypt and it had proved a happy time domestically as well as being rewarding from a professional point of view. The Egyptian Government honoured him with the award of the Order of the Nile and his colleagues staged a farewell dinner at Cairo's Turf Club. The dinner menu had a cartoon on its cover depicting Smith wearing a kilt and tarboosh and carrying a copy of *Taylor's Principles* under his arm. It was an affectionate view of a man who had achieved a great deal to advance the standing of his profession. So, Sydney and Kitty and their children left the desert sun behind them in 1928 and headed for a grey Edinburgh. One possibly small consolation was that Kitty would no longer have to buy Keating's Powder in the large quantities needed to keep Sydney clear of fleas on his excursions into Egyptian crime dens.

Returning to Britain at the beginning of April, Smith was in time to follow the trial at the Old Bailey of Frederick Guy Browne and William Henry Kennedy charged with the murder of a police constable. He had read the press reports of the shooting in an Essex country lane the previous September, while in Cairo.

It was a case in which firearms evidence played a major role and one in which the use of the comparison microscope, pioneered by Smith, represented a breakthrough in crime investigation in Britain. Robert Churchill, who had opposed his views in the Merrett case, was the expert called for the prosecution. Browne and Kennedy's conviction rested almost entirely on ballistics evidence and Churchill's biographer, Macdonald Hastings, was generous in acknowledging the stimulus which Smith had provided by developing the new techniques. For his own part, Smith said, 'I followed the case with an almost proprietary interest.'

Smith soon immersed himself in the work of the university and, although he had succeeded Harvey Littlejohn in the Chair of Forensic Medicine, he was not appointed Chief Surgeon to the Edinburgh Police. That post had been taken by Littlejohn's assistant, Dr Douglas Kerr, who made a considerable success of it. Smith was too big a man to harbour anything more than a few regrets but there is no doubt that he was disappointed at not having routine access to police work. He also missed the variety and exotic nature of the sort of cases he had encountered in Egypt. But compensation lay in the opportunity to appear as an expert witness in important criminal cases, some of which would justly be described as *causes célèbres*.

He was soon to find himself at odds again with the pre-eminent forensic expert of the day, Sir Bernard Spilsbury, when they were drawn against each other in one of the great trials of the 1920s. Spilsbury was at the peak of his impressive career. He had featured in most of the important murder cases of the century and was immensely respected by the public. But he was neither traveller nor innovator, qualities which gave Sydney Smith greater depth. What Sir Bernard possessed was single-mindedness and sureness of reputation, while Smith was largely unknown to the public and was thought of chiefly as an academic. The truth was that their experience was of equal quality but that Spilsbury had enjoyed the greater publicity.

The clash between these personalities took place at Lewes Assizes in March 1930 where Sidney Harry Fox was being tried for murder; not an ordinary murder but for the uncommon crime of killing his mother. Sixty-three-year-old Mrs Rosaline Fox perished in a fire in her bedroom at the Hotel Metropole in Margate on 22 October 1929. Her son had raised the alarm but too late to save his mother who had apparently been overcome by smoke and fumes. A verdict of accidental death was returned by a coroner's court and Mrs Fox was buried in her native Norfolk.

It was only when the dubious nature of Sidney Fox's character began to emerge that suspicion started to form. He had a record as a blackmailer and swindler and it appeared that six days before his mother died he had taken out two insurance policies on her life. As a result of enquiries by Chief Inspector Hambrook of Scotland Yard, Sidney Fox was taken into custody. Meanwhile, his mother's corpse was exhumed and a post-mortem carried out by Spilsbury. The pathologist concluded that Mrs Fox had been strangled and her son was charged with murdering her.

Sydney Smith was asked by Fox's solicitor to give evidence for the defence. After carefully examining the medical aspects of the case, he agreed to appear as an expert witness. The details of the trial for murder that ensued are covered in the preceding chapter. Apart from a man's life, what was also at stake was the reputation and integrity of Britain's foremost forensic experts. Smith was as well practised in the role of giving expert testimony as was Spilsbury, but he lacked the public acclaim. From the outset, he was intrigued by Spilsbury's post-mortem report on Mrs Fox and found it remarkable that Sir Bernard concluded from the medical evidence that she had died of 'asphyxia due to manual strangulation'. There appeared to be no external signs of injury and a complete absence of the usually unmistakable indications of strangulation. As Smith noted later, 'a person being strangled fights like mad' and, even though elderly, will struggle furiously to pull away the constricting hands.

The very nature of such a fight for life causes marks and scratches on the neck and, often, minor injuries around the mouth and nose. The unsuccessful struggle to draw air into the lungs results in blueing of the lips and ears and frothing at the mouth and nose, with the tongue frequently protruding. Moreover, there is customarily bruising of the neck muscles as the strangler tightens his grip in order to overcome the victim's struggles, with the result that the delicate internal structures of the throat are damaged. Spilsbury found none of these classic signs, yet was firm in his conclusion that death was due to strangulation.

The evidence for strangulation as cause of death was a bruise which Spilsbury had seen on the larynx of the dead woman. He had removed the tissue at post-mortem and placed it in formalin. Before Sidney Fox appeared at Sussex Assizes, Smith had the opportunity to examine the specimen in Spilsbury's laboratory at University College Hospital. The two men had met before but this was their first professional consultation or, as it turned out, confrontation.

Spilsbury produced the larynx on which he had described seeing a bruise the size of half a crown. To start with, Smith could not conceive how such a substantial internal bruise could have been inflicted without leaving external marks. But his amazement was complete when, with Spilsbury looking over his shoulder, he examined the larynx but could see no bruise at all. 'No. You can't see it now,' explained Spilsbury, 'but it was there when I exhumed the body.' Smith questioned him about the apparent disappearance of the bruise and was told that 'it became obscure before I put the larynx in formalin'. Some tight-lipped discussion ensued in which Smith expressed his incredulity that a bruise of such a size could simply disappear. He acknowledged the difficulties in differentiating between bruising and patches of putrefaction and wondered if what Spilsbury had seen was not the latter. Spilsbury listened politely but declined to accept any alternative explanation; it was a bruise and nothing more, he contended.

What would have put the matter beyond argument would have been the microscopic examination of a section of the bruised tissue. Bruising is caused by the rupture of small blood vessels which allows blood to escape into the surrounding tissue where it clots to form a patch of discolouration. Blood forced into the tissues in this way is not affected by post-mortem changes and, hence, confirmation of such bruising can be easily established microscopically. Unfortunately, Spilsbury did not take a section because, as he had explained, the bruise had become obscure before he put the larynx in preservative.

So there it was and, in court, Spilsbury, with the aid of an anatomical model of the human neck, indicated where he had found the bruise which led him to believe that Mrs Fox had been strangled. An interesting point was brought out which was that while the delicate hyoid bone in Mrs Fox's throat had apparently survived the strangler's attack, Spilsbury himself had broken it inadvertently in two places while examining it in his laboratory.

Under cross-examination by the Attorney-General, Sir William Jowitt, Sydney Smith cast doubt on the accuracy of Spilsbury's findings. Sir William seemed to be affronted that Smith dared to challenge the opinion of such a renowned figure.

'Do you suggest,' he asked, 'that Sir Bernard Spilsbury would not know the difference between discolouration due to post-mortem changes and a bruise?'

Smith, too experienced a performer to be ruffled by such exchanges, answered, 'I say no one can tell by looking at a stain whether it is a post-mortem stain or a bruise.'

The Attorney-General then asked, 'Do you say that you would never say a bruise was a bruise until you put it under a microscope?'

'No,' replied Smith, 'I should cut into it.'

Of course, he was quite correct and had Spilsbury adopted this procedure and, for good measure, taken a section for microscopic examination, the eventual confrontation of opinion need never have occurred. Thus, in a court of law where a man was on trial for his life, the cause of this victim's death for want of any confirming evidence was resolved on the basis of one doctor's observation.

In the event, Spilsbury's view won the day because of the strength of his reputation rather than the infallibility of his methods. In fairness, Mr Justice Rowlatt, in his summing up to the jury, pointed out that, 'No one can say that an individual, whatever his position and skill, is never likely to be mistaken. No one can claim for anybody infallibility.' Nevertheless, the jury believed Spilsbury and Smith did not think they would have returned a guilty verdict but for the London pathologist's evidence.

Commenting on Fox's denial of the jury's verdict that he had murdered his mother, Smith said he believed he was innocent. He would not have put the deed past him, particularly in light of the insurance he had taken out, but, despite the circumstantial evidence, he did not think he had strangled his mother. It was more likely in his view that Mrs Fox died of heart failure precipitated by the shock of waking up in a smoke-filled room. But at least one of Sidney Fox's lies was undone by Mrs Harding, wife of the Hotel Metropole's manager. In her efforts to calm the apparently distraught son who had discovered a fire in his mother's bedroom, she cradled his head and ran her fingers through his hair. Later she told her husband, 'That boy's hair is full of smoke and he never went near the room!'

Sydney Smith's place in Egypt had been taken by John Glaister who, to use the modern term, had been head-hunted for the position. Glaister was told that in Cairo he would see almost as many medico-legal cases in a week as he would see in Glasgow in a year. Certainly Egypt was a good training ground for the forensic pathologist and Smith was putting his experience of investigating murder by poisoning to good effect in a case that took him to Cornwall.

Annie Hearn, a lady in her early forties, had not enjoyed a happy life. Her husband disappeared a few days after their wedding in 1919 and despite a lack of any clear information about his fate, she took to describing herself as a widow. She lived in the Midlands with her invalid sister, Lydia Everard, who she called Minnie, until 1921, when they moved to Lewannick near Launceston in Cornwall. The move was undertaken for the benefit of Minnie, a chronic sufferer of gastric illness. Their neighbours in Trenhorne Farm were William Thomas and his wife Alice with whom they were very friendly. The two sisters and the Thomases often went out together for drinks in the countryside and, when Minnie was poorly, Alice Thomas made junkets and other delicacies for her.

This state of affairs continued for several years but in July 1930, after two or three bad bouts of gastric trouble, Minnie died. During her years of illness when she lived in Cornwall, Minnie had been treated by two doctors from the local practice and they were well aware of her condition. She was buried without fuss and her sad loss seemed to draw Annie Hearn closer to the Thomases. Their friendship continued as before and they enjoyed the occasional picnic; Annie's contribution to these outings was to provide the sandwiches.

On 18 October 1930, several months after Minnie's death, they went off on one of their afternoon excursions, equipped with sandwiches made by Annie with a tinned salmon filling. These refreshments were eaten at about 5 p.m. when they stopped for a cup of tea at a café in Bude. On the drive home, Alice Thomas was taken ill with what her husband took to be food poisoning. When they reached home, she was put to bed, suffering from vomiting and diarrhoea. A doctor was called and at around 9.30 that evening Dr Graham Saunders from Launceston attended the sick woman and diagnosed food poisoning; Annie Hearn offered to look after the patient.

Alice Thomas improved a little the following day but a relapse followed with delirium and severe cramps added to her previous symptoms. Dr Saunders now suspected arsenical poisoning and this tentative diagnosis was confirmed by a specialist called in from Plymouth. Alice Thomas died in Plymouth City Hospital on 4 November and at post-mortem a total of 0.85 grains of arsenic was found in her body. William Thomas was advised of the findings and local gossip led to speculation about Annie Hearn's relationship with the Thomases. Two days after Alice Thomas's funeral, Annie disappeared, leaving a note behind addressed to Mr Thomas:

> Goodbye. I'm going out if I can. I cannot forget that awful man and the things he said. I am <u>innocent, innocent</u>, but she is dead and it was my lunch she eat. I cannot bear it. When I'm dead they will be sure I am guilty and you at least will be cleared. May your own dear wife's presence guard and comfort you still.
>
> Yours
> A.H.

> My life is not a great thing anyhow, now dear Minnie's gone. I should be glad if you would send my love to Bessie[1] and tell her not to worry about me. I'll be all right, my conscience is clear so I'm not afraid of afterwards.

William Thomas took what appeared to be a suicide note to the police. The letter writer was traced to Looe, where her coat was found on the cliff top and one of her shoes was washed up on the beach. It looked as if Annie Hearn had indeed committed suicide. Two weeks later, the inquest on Alice Thomas concluded that she had died of arsenical poisoning and the verdict was homicide by some person or persons unknown.

On 9 December, in light of Mrs Thomas's demise due to arsenic poisoning, it was decided to exhume the body of Minnie Hearn, who had died four months previously. Dr Roche Lynch, the Home Office analyst, discovered arsenic in all the organs. An examination of the hair indicated that Minnie had been receiving arsenic for at least seven months before she died. This revelation stimulated the police to greater efforts in their hunt for Annie Hearn, not being entirely convinced that she had taken her own life. She was found after a few weeks in Torquay where she had taken work as a housekeeper using an assumed name. Her employer, Cecil Powell, recognised her from a photograph published in the *Daily*

---

1 Annie Hearn's sister who lived in Doncaster.

Mail, which offered a reward of £500[2] for information as to her whereabouts. On 18 January 1931, she was arrested and charged with the murder of Alice Thomas and her sister Minnie.

Walter West, Annie's solicitor, approached Sydney Smith and asked him to review the medical aspects of the case. Smith did not dissent from the cause of death – Alice Thomas had died as the result of arsenical poisoning – what was not clear was how and when the poison had been administered. He was convinced that the picnic sandwiches eaten on 18 October had not been the source of the arsenic, although, in all probability, the salmon had caused food poisoning. The analyst's findings made it more likely that Mrs Thomas had ingested the arsenic much nearer the time that she died.

In the case of Minnie, her medical history showed her to be a chronic sufferer of gastric troubles, although not of diarrhoea, which is one of the principal indicators of arsenical poisoning. Her own doctor had recorded death due to natural causes and Smith was inclined to agree. How then could the arsenic found in her exhumed body be explained?

When it came to poisoning by arsenic, there was probably no doctor in the British Isles more knowledgeable about the subject than Sydney Smith. He did not dispute that Dr Roche Lynch had discovered arsenic in the dead woman's muscles, nails and hair, but he was highly critical of his calculations. The analyst had reported finding a total of 0.776 of a grain in the muscles. The calculation was based on analysing a sample of tissue weighing one-eighth of an ounce and applying a standard formula to arrive at a total for the body's muscles as a whole. The sample yielded 1/6400 of a grain of arsenic which the analyst multiplied by a figure representing the mass of muscle, usually taken to be 40 per cent of the total body weight. In this instance, Roche Lynch had assumed a body weight of 80lb from which he calculated the muscle component as about 32lb.

Smith recognised immediately that 80lb is a very low body weight and the woman must obviously have been in an emaciated condition when she died. The experienced pathologist knew that in a badly wasting body, the muscles are the first to lose weight. Hence, he would have estimated the proportion of muscle to body weight in this case as nearer 15 per cent than the usual 40 per cent. In light of this, it appeared that the amount of arsenic in the body had been badly over-estimated. Of vital importance was the amount of arsenic found in the soil samples taken from the grave in Lewannick churchyard; the soil above the coffin contained 125 parts of arsenic per million and that below it, 62 parts per million. As Smith saw it, the presence of arsenic in the body would have pointed to poisoning if it had been buried in any other county of England but Cornwall. The

---

2   Cecil Powell claimed the reward and immediately turned it over to Annie Hearn's solicitor to help pay for her defence.

county was known for its tin mines and, where there is tin, there is usually arsenic to be found. Arsenic occurs naturally in the soil and is a common impurity in many metallic ores.

Smith's conclusion was that, while arsenic was undoubtedly found in the body of Annie Hearn's sister, he doubted that its presence was an indicator of cause of death. He believed she had died of natural causes and that the arsenic had most likely infiltrated her corpse from the soil surrounding the grave in which she had lain for over four months. As for Alice Thomas, the indications were that the famous salmon sandwiches might have precipitated the food poisoning which she undoubtedly suffered but that the arsenic was administered after that time. In other words, the two cases provided less than conclusive evidence of Annie Hearn's guilt and that was the substance of Smith's report to her solicitor.

Annie Hearn's trial had been fixed in the legal calendar to start on 15 June 1931 at Bodmin Assizes. In his reply to Walter West, Smith had mentioned that he would not be available to attend the trial owing to the pressures of his university teaching programme. He changed his mind when he received an urgent telegram requesting a meeting with Norman Birkett, the distinguished lawyer who had taken on the task of defending Annie Hearn. Birkett told him that he might not call him to give evidence but that he would like him by his side in court. By drawing out the points that suited his argument in his cross-examination of the prosecution witnesses, and by calling Annie Hearn as the sole witness for the defence, Birkett secured the right to address the jury after the Crown had concluded its case.

The prosecution case took six days and, with help from Smith who passed him notes on the forensic aspects of the evidence, Birkett began to demolish its credibility. Concerning the exhumation of the bodies at Lewannick, he suggested that in an area distinguished for the mineral content of its soil, arsenic could readily have contaminated the exhumed corpse and open specimen jars from dust in the churchyard. 'Am I right in saying,' he asked the doctor who carried out the post-mortem, 'that a piece of soil, so small that you could hold it between your fingers, and dropped on to the body would make every single calculation wrong?'

'Yes,' came the answer.

Later in the proceedings, sixty-year-old Herbert du Parcq, leading counsel for the Crown, collapsed and was taken from the courtroom. The way the trial had been proceeding, this might have been seen by some superstitious members of a Cornish jury as a warning from the Almighty not to convict an innocent woman. Certainly Mr Justice Roche was at pains to point out that Mr du Parcq's indisposition was not something of which a mystery should be made.

In any event, Birkett had taken a firm hold on the trial and he dealt severely with Dr Roche Lynch when he said he had never attended one living patient suffering from arsenical poisoning, 'yet he speaks of symptoms with the same confidence that he spoke on other matters.'

'Let the cobbler stick to his last . . .' was his stinging rebuttal.

Having weakened the prosecution case regarding the arsenical poisoning of Annie Hearn's sister, Birkett turned his attention to the poisoning of Mrs Thomas. The vehicle for administering the poison was alleged to be the salmon in the sandwiches made by Annie and the poison was supposed to be weedkiller which she had bought four years previously.

Smith had done his homework on this aspect of the case knowing that the Arsenic Act of 1851 required arsenical preparations to be coloured with indigo, he had little doubt that when powdered arsenic was sprinkled onto a sandwich, the filling would become discoloured. Roche Lynch had estimated that about 14.3 grains of weedkiller would have been used and the implication was that Annie Hearn added the poison to the sandwiches a few hours before they were eaten. To be absolutely sure of his ground, Smith carried out an experiment with tinned salmon and weedkiller. Within half an hour, his sandwiches thus prepared were stained a bluish-purple.

Armed with this information, Birkett was able to test Roche Lynch in cross-examination. 'If you put fourteen grains (of arsenic) in a moist sandwich and carried it for hours,' he asked, 'is it not inevitable that the sandwich would be discoloured and blue?'

'I have not tried it,' answered Roche Lynch, adding rather unwisely, 'but my opinion, for what it is worth, is that it would not.' Birkett could easily have demolished the witness but he chose not to, believing, correctly, that he was winning his case in any event.

When he discussed the content of his closing speech with Sydney Smith, Birkett acknowledged the religious nature of the Cornish people. He said he would illustrate the paradox of the loving care which Annie Hearn gave to her sister with the contention that she was also poisoning her, by quoting from The New Testament. The gospel according to St John contains the passage, 'in my Father's house are many mansions: if it were not so, I would have told you. I go to prepare a place for you.' Birkett changed his mind when he heard that the jury on its last night together, which happened to be a Sunday, was offered the choice of attending church or going for a drive and elected for the latter. 'Ah! There go my Father's Mansions,' he remarked to Smith.

In a powerful closing address, he asked the jury, by its verdict, to send Annie Hearn 'back into the sunlight away from the shadows which have haunted her for so long'. They did just that by bringing in a 'Not Guilty' verdict. Three weeks after she was acquitted, Annie Hearn wrote to Sydney Smith thanking him for putting aside important engagements 'to come to Bodmin and help to save a life, my life.' Annie Hearn disappeared into obscurity but, despite her acquittal, local gossip persisted in believing that she was discharged, less on account of her innocence than because of Herbert du Parcq's collapse and Norman Birkett's masterly defence of which Sydney Smith was the chief architect.

Controversy seemed to surround many of the cases with which Smith became involved. Hard on the heels of the Hearn trial came a death by strangling which brought him and Spilsbury together again, not in confrontation as in the Fox trial, but both arguing in the defence of a man charged with murder. As Smith put it, 'It was the first time we had been colleagues in a case – and it was also the last.'

Peter Queen was a thirty-one-year-old clerk who worked in his father's bookmaker's business in Glasgow. In the early hours of Saturday, 21 November 1931, he walked into one of the city's police stations; he placed two house keys on the desk and said, 'Go to 539 Dumbarton Road, I think you will find my wife dead.' Two constables were despatched to the address given. In the bedroom of Queen's two-room apartment, they found the pyjama-clad body of a woman lying on the bed with a piece of cord tied around her neck.

Chrissie Gall, aged twenty-eight, was not Queen's wife but she had been living with him for several months. She lay with the bedclothes pulled up over her chest, her left arm was outside the blankets and her right arm was underneath. One of the policemen loosened the rope around her neck which had been pulled tight in a half-knot. There were no signs of a struggle having taken place; everything about the room, and particularly the bed, was neat and tidy. There was no doubting that Chrissie Gall had been strangled and Peter Queen was charged with her murder.

Strangulation was confirmed as the cause of death by the pathologist carrying out the post-mortem who discovered the usual signs of asphyxia in the internal organs. The ligature around the dead woman's neck had been pulled sufficiently tight to create a groove in her flesh and the cricoid cartilage in her throat was broken. Not surprisingly, this led to the conclusion that her death was homicidal.

Chrissie Gall's personal history was highly relevant in this case. She had only ever worked 'in service' and had developed a weakness for drinking. When she met Peter Queen, he tried to wean her away from alcohol; at the time, he was separated from his wife, who was being treated for chronic alcoholism. The couple moved in together in December 1930 and, with the aid of friends, Queen sought to combat her drunkenness. She was subject to bouts of depression and, in the presence of friends, had threatened to commit suicide by drowning herself; 'making a hole in the Clyde', as she termed it. On another occasion she attempted to gas herself and spoke also of hanging herself or of taking an overdose.

During the two days prior to her death, Chrissie was in a state of almost continuous inebriation. She spent the final day of her life in bed, sleeping and being cared for by friends who tried to persuade her to eat and drink something non-alcoholic. She was awake when the friends left at about 10.45 but a little over four hours later Queen reported that she was dead.

Smith and Spilsbury examined the bedroom at Dumbarton Road and together considered their stance on the likely cause of death. The natural position of the body with upper denture still in place, the undisturbed bedclothes and tidiness of the room all indicated a lack of struggle and went against murder. The physical signs on the body lacked the telling force of murderous strangulation. There was no bruising in the deeper structures of the neck which indicated that only a small degree of force had been used. This was consistent with the half-knot which had been used to pull the ligature tight around the neck. Stranglers usually employ considerable force, first to overcome the struggles of their victim and then, when a ligature is involved, to prevent the knot slipping.

Spilsbury concluded, 'It was a suicide.' Smith agreed. 'Certainly there isn't much to suggest murder,' he said, adding, 'I have never seen a case of homicide by strangulation in an adult in which there were so few signs.' He was still concerned though over the half-knot and he wondered if it would have kept tight enough to cause asphyxia after Chrissie Gall had lost consciousness and released her grip on the ends of the cord. Spilsbury partially satisfied him on this point after examining the cord, part of a clothesline, under a microscope. It could be seen that the fibres were roughened at the point where the ends of the cord crossed over and bit into one another.

The trial of Peter Queen was held in Glasgow on 5 January 1932 and lasted five days. There were a number of unsatisfactory aspects of the prosecution's case. It was alleged that Queen's declaration to the police, 'I think I have killed her', was as good as a confession. It was due to close questioning by the Lord Justice Clerk, Lord Alness, that it emerged the police had not made a written record of Queen's remarks. The accused man, when he reported Chrissie's death, claimed he had said, 'Don't think I have killed her'. There was an obvious world of difference between the two versions. Furthermore, the doctors who had carried out the post-mortem neglected to carry out an analysis of either the blood or the stomach contents. This was particularly unfortunate as the murder allegation rested on the assumption that the victim had been too drunk to resist. In the absence of proof of alcohol in the dead woman's system this remained at best an assumption.

The experts for the prosecution, including Dr Andrew Allison, Professor of Medical Jurisprudence at Glasgow, contended that the appearance of the body did not indicate suicide. Against this view was the weight of Spilsbury's evidence, supported by Sydney Smith, that self-strangulation was entirely consistent with the circumstances of the woman's death. Although Smith tended towards the suicide explanation, he was not entirely convinced. The case was very much on the border-line but not for Spilsbury, whose lack of hesitation in giving his opinions 'took my breath away', said Smith later. In the event, the jury rejected the Scottish formula for dealing with borderline cases – the Not Proven verdict – and found Peter Queen guilty. As Smith recorded in due course in his memoirs, '. . . in the only case where Spilsbury and I were in pretty complete agreement, the jury believed neither of us.'

Although sentenced to death, Queen was reprieved following an impressive public petition raised on his behalf by the citizens of Glasgow. He worked in his former occupation of bookmaker's clerk when he was released from prison until he died in 1958. Smith believed there was insufficient evidence to justify Queen's conviction and admitted that suicide by strangulation was not a common phe-nomenon although there were a number of recorded incidents. Indeed he came across another case of self-strangulation a short while after Queen's conviction. The victim was a forty-five-year-old spinster who suffered from depression. She died by a combination of smothering and strangulation; a handkerchief was found inside her mouth blocking the air passages and a scarf had been tied tightly around her throat. Like Chrissie Gall, she had threatened suicide when friends were present and the scene of her death was marked by a similar lack of distur-bance. The advent of the nylon stocking and of materials with high elasticity have made self-strangulation more feasible. A pre-knotted ligature can be stretched over the head and, once around the neck, the material contracts to its original shape, thereby exerting a powerful constriction effect.

Smith's next encounter with Spilsbury was less congenial. The two pathologists appeared on opposite sides of the fence in a controversial case involving the repu-tation of a fellow doctor. Abortion was not a subject discussed in polite society in the 1930s and any doctor accused of carrying out a criminal abortion faced a very serious charge indeed. In October 1933, Dr Avarne, a member of the surgical staff of the General Hospital at St Helier in Jersey, travelled to Edinburgh to consult Smith on a professional matter – he had been charged with carrying out a crimi-nal abortion and was due to face trial the next month.

The circumstances involved Dr Avarne's friendship with a hotel proprietor in Jersey who asked him to advise on the delicate matter of his young mistress's pregnancy. The twenty-eight-year-old woman had been pregnant in 1926 when the putative father gave her money to have the baby in England. When she told him in May 1933 that she was pregnant again, he denied responsibility but sug-gested she see Dr Avarne who was a personal friend.

From the moment that Avarne agreed to see the woman, disaster loomed for the doctor. He first saw her on 27 May when she was eight and a half weeks pregnant and at a second consultation a month later, prescribed nothing more potent than a bromide sedative. On 21 July, complaining of pain and loss of blood, she was admitted to the Jersey nursing home run by Sister Le Feuvre. Dr Avarne took charge of the patient, explaining the circumstances to the Sister and advising her that he might need to carry out an examination under anaesthetic on the following day. The doctor attempted to induce abortion and, when this failed, carried out a second operation to remove the foetus with instruments. This also failed. After an interval of twenty-four hours, the patient's general condition deteriorated and she experienced rigor accompanied by a high temperature. During the evening of 27 July, her child was born dead. All efforts to contact Dr Avarne failed but Sister Le Feuvre's anxiety was relieved when another doctor called at the nursing home to deal with a different patient. Dr Bentlif was pressed into service and when the woman recovered consciousness, she told him what she described as 'the whole truth'. This was to the effect that she had neither pain nor haemorrhage when admitted to the nursing home but made these complaints on the instructions of Dr Avarne who had agreed to terminate her pregnancy. Dr Bentlif, without waiting to contact Avarne, called the police.

The woman made a statement to the police which she later repeated to Dr Blampied, the police surgeon, when he called at the nursing home. The foetus and the placenta were put in specimen jars for further examination by doctors who agreed that there were no indications of softening of the tissues which would be expected if the baby had died in the womb. This boded ill for Dr Avarne, now under arrest, as it appeared that he had indeed carried out a criminal abortion. The patient made a complete recovery but her doctor now faced criminal proceedings.

Spilsbury was called in to advise the Crown and, after examining the pathological material, confirmed the views of the local doctors that there was no softening of the tissues. But Dr Avarne maintained the foetus was dead when his patient was admitted to the nursing home, hence its removal was vital to protect the life of the mother. It was at this point that Sydney Smith entered the contest and he enlisted the help of an Edinburgh colleague, Professor Murray Drennan, of the Pathology Department. They made microscopic sections from the tissues of the foetus and placenta from which they concluded that signs of softening or maceration were present. Furthermore, there were indications of haemorrhage in the placenta and, thus, strong arguments in their view to support the correctness of Dr Avarne's diagnosis.

If it could be proved satisfactorily that the woman was carrying a dead child, the case against her doctor simply evaporated. Smith agreed to appear on Dr Avarne's behalf but, realising his lack of experience in gynaecology, decided to enlist expert help. He secured the services of Dr Aleck Bourne, a leading London gynaecologist, who examined the pathological material in the presence of both Smith and Spilsbury. Bourne's opinion was that the child had been dead for several days before birth. These defence arguments, including the microscopic sections, were demonstrated to Spilsbury but he declined to shift his opinion.

Dr Avarne appeared before the Bailiff of Jersey sitting with ten magistrates and a jury of twenty-four. It was a formidable, if quaint, array of legal presence. The proceedings derived from the island's Norman French history and Sydney Smith was surprised to see all the witnesses sworn in together, followed by their examination by the Attorney-General without the formality of any opening statement. The rules allowed a verdict to be brought in on a two-thirds majority.

Three of Jersey's senior medical men gave it as their opinion that neither the foetus nor the placenta demonstrated any indication of maceration that could be taken to show the child was dead in the womb. Sir Bernard Spilsbury lent his weight to this view, and said there had been no haemorrhaging prior to the woman being admitted to the nursing home and that the foetus died during the second operation carried out on her by Dr Avarne. Spilsbury threw his customary astuteness to the wind when he allowed himself to be drawn into answering questions outside his field. He criticised the clinical treatment carried out by Dr Avarne which he said was not appropriate for the circumstances. He was to pay the penalty for this somewhat arrogant approach later on during the trial.

A number of the doctors appearing as prosecution witnesses spoke highly of Dr Avarne, praising his abilities as a surgeon and casting not the slightest doubt on his past professional conduct. Admiring appraisals of the accused doctor came from the defence witnesses, one of whom declared that hundreds of people in Jersey had cause to thank Dr Avarne for his medical skills. Such fulsome testimonials were heart-warming but amounted to very little when measured against the medical background of the case. Spilsbury had said his piece but the star-performer was yet to come.

Smith's suggestion to invite testimony for the defence from a leading gynaecologist was shrewd. He and Dr Aleck Bourne had thoroughly prepared their evidence and they appeared as final witnesses in the trial. Their conclusion was simply that the child was dead within the mother's womb before Dr Avarne operated on her. Bourne had no doubts at all that the Jersey doctor had acted properly and implemented the correct treatment. He dismissed contemptuously the suggestion that a criminal abortion had been carried out; it was, he said, 'asking one to believe an almost impossible thing that Dr Avarne would have attempted to perform a criminal abortion at the period he had.' He also reserved some vitriol for Spilsbury's opinion on the case. Counsel asked him if he considered the evidence given by Sir Bernard, who enjoyed a worldwide reputation, to be regarded as unbelievable. He replied, 'I have the greatest respect and admiration for Sir Bernard when he speaks as a pathologist, but when he dares to give an opinion about the treatment of a living woman I would regard it with contempt.' These were strong words and of a kind rarely addressed to Spilsbury, but on this occasion at least, they were merited, for the London pathologist admitted he had not been medically involved with a case of pregnancy for twenty years.

Dr Avarne was found 'Not Guilty' to cheers from the public gallery and from a crowd of several thousand outside the court. An obviously admired physician had his reputation restored to him and justice was done. There was a great deal of quiet satisfaction in the outcome for Sydney Smith. In his patient way, he had spiked Spilsbury's guns, not with rhetoric or argument but with superior science. One of the sad aspects of professional life which came out of the Jersey abortion case was the bitterness and relish with which opposing factions in the medical hierarchy fought each other. This had been a factor in bringing the initial charge against Dr Avarne. Sadder still was that the same sense of professional rivalry should prevail amongst the aristocrats of the profession. Spilsbury, who would later have harsh appraisals written about him by his peers, was also sufficiently small minded to mete out his own petty retribution. Whereas Spilsbury, Smith and Bourne had voyaged together amicably across to Jersey from the mainland before the trial, their return was less friendly. They travelled on the same boat but Spilsbury would not speak to the pair who had bested him in court.

Sydney Smith had a knack for accepting difficult and controversial cases; he also liked the challenge of investigations which nudged the frontiers of forensic knowledge. One such case was the murder of a child in Aberdeen in 1934. On 20 April, eight-year-old Helen Priestly went missing from her home in Urquhart Road. The child had returned home after school at about 12.15 p.m. and ate lunch with her mother. Afterwards, at about 1.30 p.m., she was sent to the bakery a few minutes walk from home to buy a loaf of bread. Helen was due to go back to school in King Street at 2 p.m. and when she failed to return home by 1.50, her mother decided to walk round to the bakery to hurry her up. There she learned that her daughter had been and gone at least a quarter of an hour previously. Mrs Priestly next went to the school and, there, her anxieties deepened, for Helen was not in her class.

By 5 p.m. the disappearance of Helen Priestly had been reported to the police and officers were making preliminary enquiries. John Priestly and his wife, aided by neighbours, drove around the district on what turned out to be a wet, windy night, searching for their only child. The police concentrated their efforts on the four-storey tenements which lined Urquhart Road. Washhouses, coal sheds and passages were systematically searched and, around 5 a.m. the next day, Helen Priestly's body was discovered almost on her own doorstep. A man taking part in the search entered the tenement and noticed a sack lying in a recess under the stairs on the ground floor immediately beneath the Priestlys' flat. Closer inspection in the grey dawn light revealed a child's foot protruding from the opening of the sack.

Dr Robert Richards, the police surgeon, was called to the scene. He noticed immediately that the sack was completely dry which indicated it had not been brought in from outdoors where it had been raining for several hours. After photographs had been taken, the doctor removed the body from the sack. The child was fully clothed except for her knickers and her body was cold and rigid. Although, when found, she lay on her right side, post-mortem lividity caused by blood draining to the bottom of the vessels on her left side clearly indicated she had been moved. Cinder particles in the sack had stuck to the girl's teeth and hair and there were traces of vomit around her mouth. It was also apparent that she had suffered severe injuries in the genital area. Word soon passed round that Helen Priestly had been raped.

The body was removed to the mortuary for a full post-mortem which was carried out by Professor Theodore Shennan, Professor of Pathology at Aberdeen University, assisted by Dr Richards. The dead child's stomach contained the undigested meat and potatoes which she had eaten for lunch at 12.30. From the small amount of digestion which had occurred, the doctors were able to make a reasonably accurate assessment of the time of death, which they put at around 2 p.m.

Helen's neck bore the evidence of an attempt at strangulation; there were bruises on her throat and vomitus in the windpipe and bronchial passages. Death from asphyxia was thus the fairly obvious cause of death. Examination of the injuries to the girl's sexual organs presented a more difficult diagnostic puzzle. The tissues of the vagina had been severely torn, resulting in considerable loss of blood, and there was a penetrating wound from the vagina into the intestinal wall. These injuries had been inflicted before death and it was quite clear that they had not been caused by an assault amounting to rape. It was far more likely that a sharp object had been thrust into the vaginal opening. The doctors used ultraviolet illumination in a search for semen but could find no traces. The true nature of the injuries slowly became apparent – they constituted a crude, simulated rape, with the implication that either a man or a woman could have inflicted them.

Police officers began the painstaking task of interviewing all the residents in the tenement block in which Helen Priestly's body had been found. They knew now that they need not restrict their enquiries to the male occupants of the building. On 25 April, officers knocked on the door of the ground-floor flat occupied by Alexander Donald, his wife Jeannie and their nine-year-old daughter, also called Jeannie. The Donalds were not a particularly sociable family, keeping themselves to themselves apart from church going and encouraging their daughter in her ambition to be a dancer. Young Jeannie Donald occasionally played with Helen Priestly, but there was a history of quarrelling between them.

Alexander Donald, a barber by trade, was, uncharacteristically for that calling, a dull, taciturn man. He answered questions in a matter-of-fact manner, explaining that he had heard the commotion outside their flat when Helen Priestly's body was found. He and his wife were in bed at the time but they did not feel sufficiently curious to investigate what was happening, even after Mrs Donald had remarked, 'Do you hear? That's Mrs Joss's voice. She's screaming that the child was raped.' The use of the word 'rape' struck a chord with Detective Inspector Taylor, for he was sure in his own mind that only Dr Richards had used that term and not in a tone of voice that could have been overheard inside a nearby flat.

The following day, detectives returned to the Donalds' home. After further questioning, permission was sought to carry out a search of the house. Some stains were found in a kitchen cupboard which, on preliminary testing, proved to be blood. Alexander and Jeannie Donald were arrested and charged with murdering Helen Priestly. He said he was 'not guilty' and his wife stated, 'I did not do that.' Shortly after midnight, they were escorted through a hostile crowd to a waiting police van and driven to the police station.

Although laboratory tests on the stains found in the Donalds' house failed to confirm them as blood, the couple remained in custody. Five days after they were arrested, the Procurator Fiscal asked Sydney Smith to lend his forensic skills to an investigation that was beginning to founder on Alexander Donald's undoubted alibi and his wife's vehement denials. Donald was released after six weeks when it was shown conclusively that, at the time the murder was committed, he was at work in his barbershop. Jeannie Donald's alibi did not stand up well to close scrutiny and she continued to be regarded with suspicion. Smith's job was to determine whether or not that suspicion had any foundation. He confirmed what everyone now believed, which was that there was no question of rape having being committed – simulated rape perhaps – and that there was a degree of circumstantial evidence pointing towards Jeannie Donald. An interesting item of gossip picked up by the police was that the dead girl did not like Mrs Donald and was in the habit of calling her 'Coconut'. This hardly seemed sufficient provocation to commit murder but the investigators' minds were busy constructing theories.

Smith knew that what was required was trace evidence linking Helen Priestly to the place where she was killed. He began looking carefully at the sack in which the body was found. It was a commonplace jute sack with the letters BOSS printed on it in red. Enquiries identified it as part of a consignment of cereals originating in Canada. Nine other sacks were found in the Donalds' house but none with the BOSS identification. It was a matter of interest that the sack in which Helen's body was found had a hole in one corner, perhaps enabling it to be hung from a nail or a hook – the Donalds' sacks all had a similar hole.

Inside the sack was a quantity of washed cinders, ordinary household fluff and a number of hairs. Starting with the cinders, Smith ascertained that Mrs Donald was the only householder in the tenement in the habit of washing her cinders, indeed traces of this practice were found in the sink trap in her kitchen.

The cinders found in the sack were examined microscopically and compared with cinders taken from all the houses in the tenement. In addition, samples were sent for specialist examination by X-ray, spectrographic and micro-chemical methods. All these tests proved inconclusive.

Smith next turned his attention to the hairs found in the sack, some of which were human and others animal. The possibility of using hair as a means of personal identification had long intrigued forensic scientists. It was John Glaister, Smith's successor in Egypt, who had made a special study of this subject and written the definitive work on it in 1931. It was to Glaister that he turned for help in the Aberdeen child murder investigation.

The human hairs in the sack did not belong to the dead child, they were coarser and of a different colour. The hairs were also irregular in contour, indicating they had been subjected to some form of artificial waving. Samples of Jeannie Donald's hair were obtained from her in prison – they showed identical characteristics to those found in the sack. Smith knew, of course, that while this comparison was significant it would not stand up as evidence without corroboration. He sent all the hair samples to Glaister for a second opinion and on 30 May Helen Priestly's body was exhumed in order that hair samples could be taken from it. The two professors of forensic pathology spent many hours bent over their microscopes in Edinburgh and Glasgow examining hair samples.

Having exhausted the hair samples, Sydney Smith next turned his microscope on the household fluff found in the sack. This material which collects in all homes is usually a composite of common fibres deriving from clothing and the furnishings of the house. There will also be dust and other materials brought into the house from outside on shoes and clothing. This unprepossessing material is a microcosm of a household's characteristics. The little balls of household fluff found in the BOSS sack contained over 200 separately identifiable materials. These ranged from wool, cotton, linen and silk fibres to cat and rabbit hairs.

Smith's intention was to compare the content of the fluff in the sack with that of fluff taken from the Donalds' house. If the two materials showed a high degree of correspondence, it was likely they originated from the same source. Using the comparison microscope which he had so successfully developed in Egypt for examining bullets side-by-side, Smith now started to compare his slides, each containing a particular type of fibre teased out of the household fluff samples.

Twenty-five different fibres were found to match completely between the two sources and there were no similar comparisons with samples taken from the other houses in the tenement. 'The absolute matching of so many different fibres from the two sources', said Smith, 'was, in my opinion, good evidence that the fluff in the sack was derived from the Donalds' house.' During the six weeks following the Donalds' arrests, their house was searched many times and any trace or stain that might be of value to the investigators was studied. Human blood was found on a number of articles of clothing, on two newspapers dated 19 April, the day before Helen Priestly's disappearance, and on a scrubbing brush and house flannels kept under the kitchen sink. The bloodstains were of Group O blood, the same as the dead child. This was not significant in itself, as 46 per cent of the population fall into Group O, but Jeannie Donald belonged to a different group. Another connecting link was provided by microbiological evidence. The same rare species of intestinal bacteria that were present on the dead child's blood-stained clothing as a result of her severe internal injuries, were also found on one of the house flannels in the Donalds' house. Again, this was highly indicative of a common source and Smith's hunch about this was confirmed by Professor Thomas Mackie, bacteriologist at Edinburgh University.

Smith was aware that Helen Priestly had an enlarged thymus gland in her neck which gives rise to a condition known as *status lymphaticus*. He bore this in mind when he reconstructed his version of the events which led to Helen Priestly's death. Enlargement of the lymphatic tissue can predispose a child to loss of consciousness when subjected to a sudden shock. Smith believed that the young girl, returning from the errand set by her mother, had seen Jeannie Donald and taunted her, as she had done before, with the shout of 'Coconut'. Infuriated, Jeannie Donald grabbed at the child and roughed her up, during the course of which, due to her enlarged thymus gland, Helen reacted by falling unconscious. Terrified that she had killed the girl, Donald dragged her into the house and decided to fake a rape attack by inserting an instrument of some sort into her vagina. The pain caused the child to regain consciousness, adding to Donald's panic and provoking her into strangling Helen. When she had regained her composure, Jeannie Donald began to clean up and, as a temporary measure, put the dead body in the cinder box which was kept under the kitchen sink. In due course, the body was transferred to the BOSS sack and put into the passage under the stairs outside the house where it was found later. What she had not accounted for in her otherwise careful clean-up operations was the incriminating nature of trace evidence transferred from her house into the sack containing her victim.

Jeannie Donald was tried for murder at Edinburgh on 16 July 1934 and after hearing the evidence of 164 witnesses, the jury brought in a guilty verdict. Donald, who had maintained an impassive stance throughout the trial, collapsed when the verdict was announced. The sentence of death passed on her was commuted to one of penal servitude, which Smith believed was right. In his view, she had no intention of killing the child, and merely wanted to frighten her. He suggested before the trial that the plea might be reduced to one of culpable homicide, a Scottish plea similar to manslaughter in the English courts. The defence would not entertain this idea, apparently preferring to go all out for a 'not guilty' verdict; 'they underestimated the medical and scientific evidence,' wrote Smith.

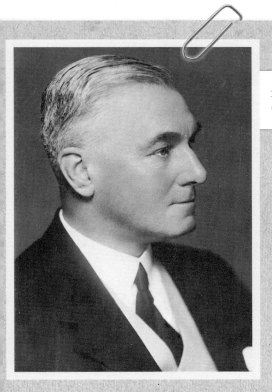

1   Sir Bernard Spilsbury.
(National Portrait Gallery)

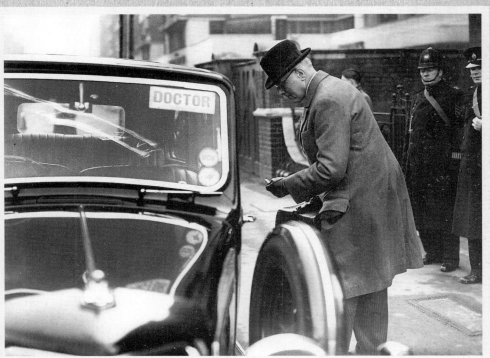

2   Pathologist on call. Spilsbury arrives at the inquest on
Sir Michael O'Dwyer. 1940. (Topical Press)

Mark ♂ ? Unknown   Fire in Motor Car.   I
10.11. ... .30.   Rex v A H Rouse

Northampton Body. Severely burned Top of head & vault of Skull completely destroyed. Brain expired shrunken & burned on top. Skin of face destroyed & ears. Faint deep burning of front of neck + of chest whole chest wall destroyed in front & front of heart + lungs exposed & partly burned Skin of abdominal wall destroyed in front but abdomen not opened. Ext genitals destroyed + Skin of Limbs. Forearms + hands completely destroyed + bone of each upper arm quite half burnt

3   Spilsbury's post-mortem record card in the Rouse case, 1930. (Gaute Archive)

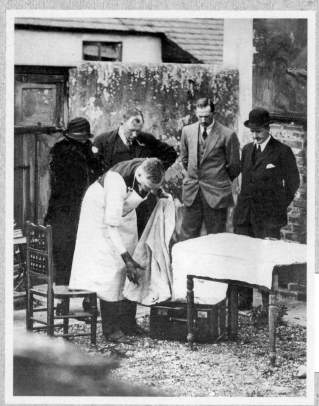

4   Spilsbury at the scene of the Crumbles murder, 1924. (London News Agency)

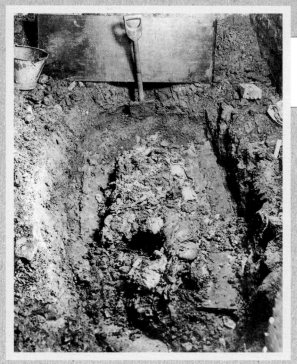

31, Marlborough Hill,
St. John's Wood, N.W.
19th January, 1922.

Dear Sir,

re Mrs. K.M. Armstrong deceased.

I enclose a report giving the results of my investigations in the above case.   I may have further information regarding the fauna of the dead body but it will not modify my conclusions.

Lest it should seem strange for flies to be about in February Dr. Hincks told me when we saw the animals that he had noticed the large numbers of flies in the sick room and that he commented upon it.

Believe me,

Yours faithfully,

(Sgd)   BERNARD H. SPILSBURY.

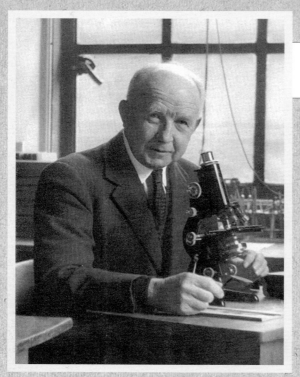

7   Sir Sydney Smith. (Harrap)

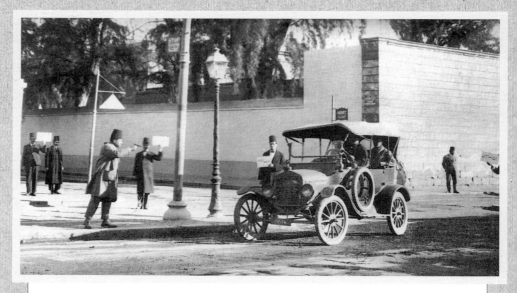

8   Reconstruction of the murder of the Sirdar, 1924. (Harrap)

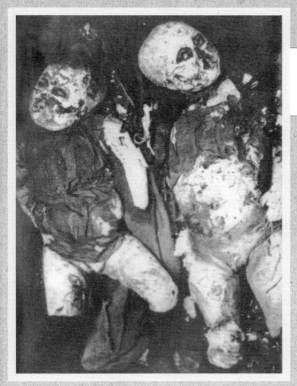

9 Children's bodies found at Hopetoun Quarry, 1913. (Harrap)

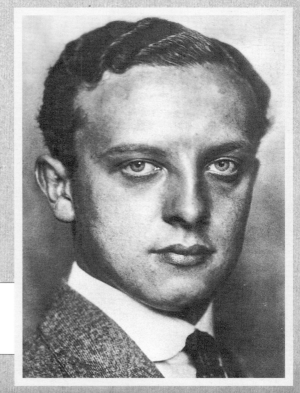

10 Sidney Fox, who murdered his mother in 1929. (Gaute Archive)

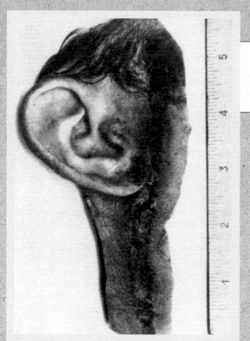

11 Bertha Merrett's ear featured as a murder exhibit in 1926. (Gaute Archive)

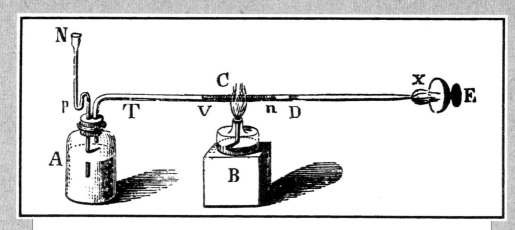

12 Marsh Test apparatus. (Gaute Archive)

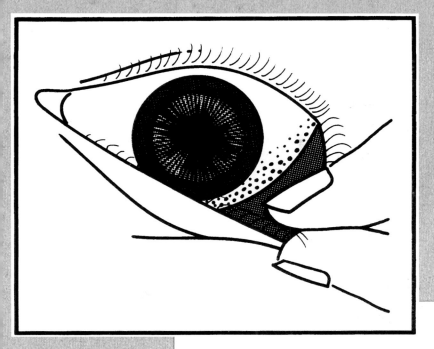

13   Petechial haemorrhages in the eye.
(Author's collection)

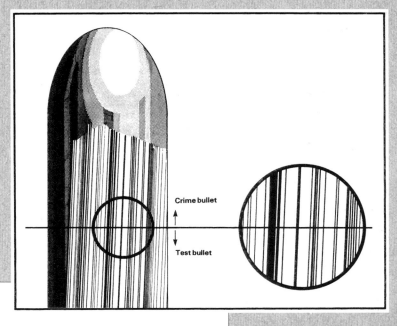

Crime bullet

Test bullet

14   Comparing striation marks on bullets.
(Author's collection)

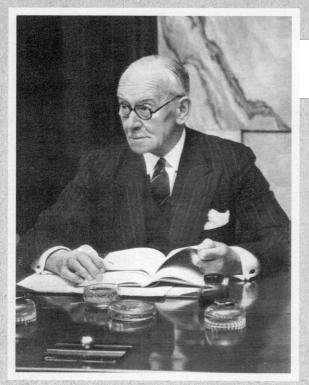

15 Professor John Glaister. (Hutchinson)

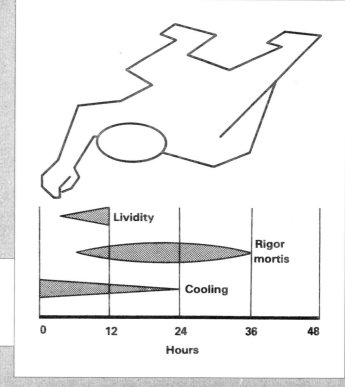

16 Calculating the time of death. (Author's collection)

Lividity

Rigor mortis

Cooling

0   12   24   36   48

Hours

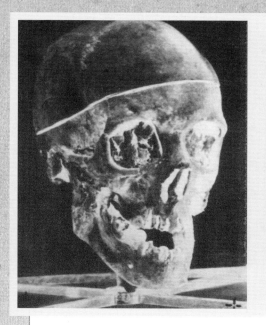
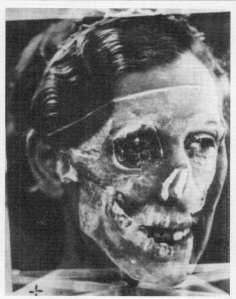

17   Isabella Ruxton's skull. (Gaute Archive)

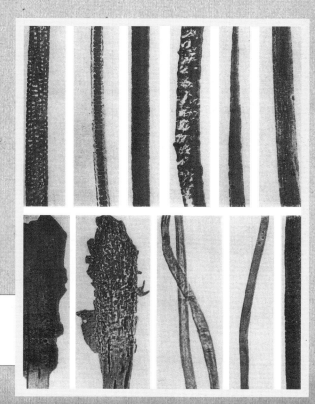

18   Comparison of
hairs and fibres.
(Gaute Archive)

Lancaster.
14.10.35.

I killed Mrs Ruxton in a fit of
temper because I thought she had
been with a man. I was Mad at
the time. Mary Rogerson was present at
the time, I had to Kill her.

B Ruxton.

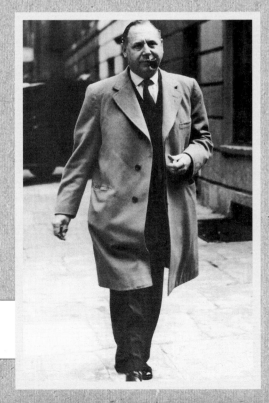

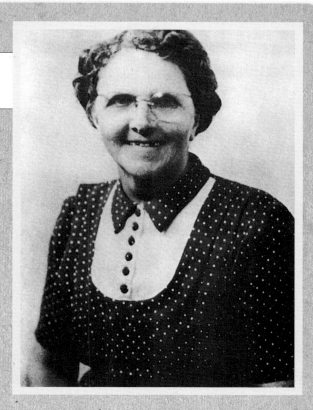

21 Sarah Jane Harvey.
(Press Association)

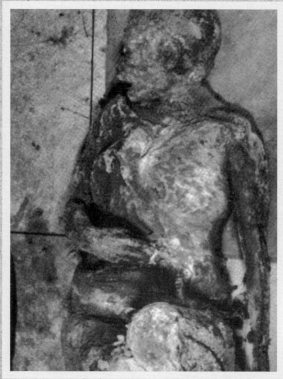

22 The Mummy of Rhyl.
(Press Association)

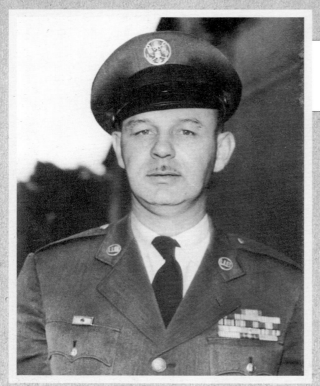

23 Staff Sergeant Marcus Marymont. (Press Association)

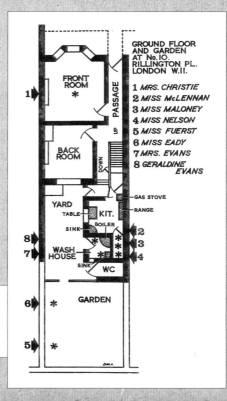

GROUND FLOOR AND GARDEN AT No. 10. RILLINGTON PL. LONDON W.11.

1 MRS. CHRISTIE
2 MISS McLENNAN
3 MISS MALONEY
4 MISS NELSON
5 MISS FUERST
6 MISS EADY
7 MRS. EVANS
8 GERALDINE EVANS

FRONT ROOM

BACK ROOM

PASSAGE

UP

DOWN

GAS STOVE

YARD

TABLE

KIT.

RANGE

SINK

BOILER

WASH HOUSE

SINK

WC

GARDEN

24 Floor plan of 10 Rillington Place and where the bodies were found. (Michael Joseph)

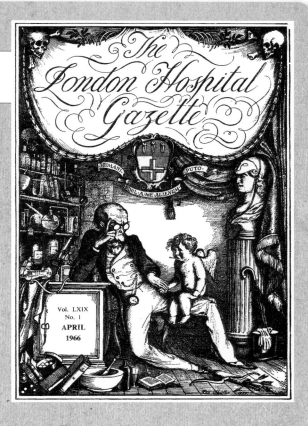

25 The *London Hospital Gazette*, 1966. (LHG)

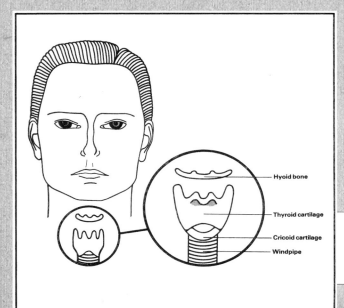

26 The human larynx. (Author's collection)

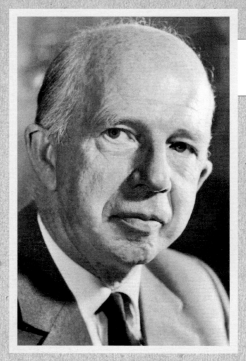

27 Professor Keith Simpson. (Harrap)

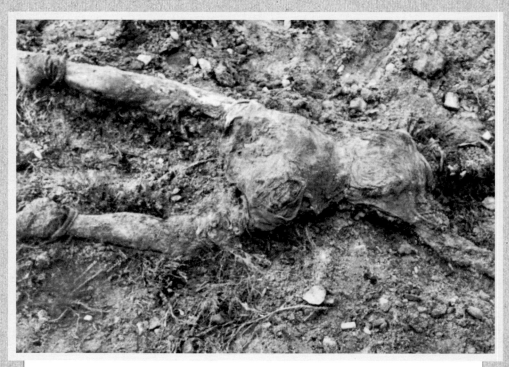

28 The body of the 'Wigwam Girl', found on Hankley Common in 1942. (Harrap)

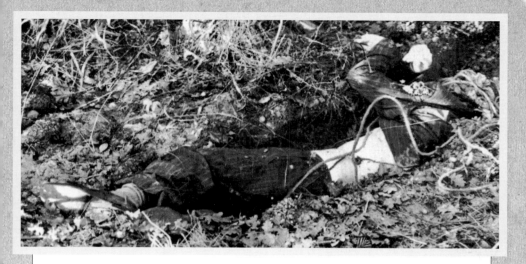

29   The 'Chalkpit Murder' victim, 1946. (Harrap)

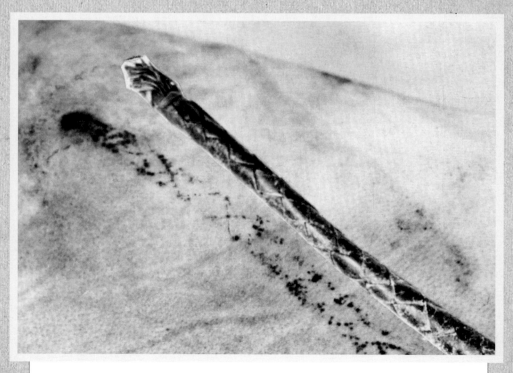

30   The diamond-weave whip in the Heath case, 1946. (Harrap)

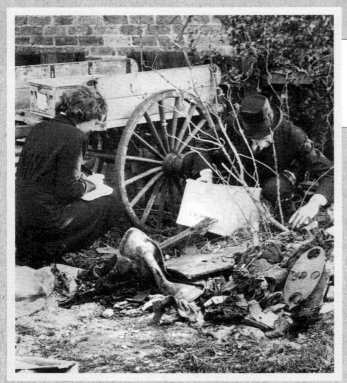

31 Sifting through the debris at George Haigh's workshop, 1949. (Harrap)

32 George Haigh's order for sulphuric acid, 1949. (Harrap)

UNION GROUP ENGINEERING

THIS NUMBER MUST BE QUOTED

ORDER

CRAWLEY   CROYDON
PUTNEY   WIMBLEDON
GENERAL ENGINEERING. SMALL REPETITION.
GAUGE MAKERS TO M.O.S. and I.G.A.

FROM THE TECHNICAL LIAISON OFFICER
ONSLOW COURT HOTEL
LONDON, S.W.7.
TELEPHONE: KENSINGTON 6300

To Alfred White Son Ltd,   16 Feby.   1949
28 Dallington St
Goswell Road E.C.1.

Please supply, Carriage Paid, to the address given below, the undermentioned goods:

1 Carbony Com H₂SO₄.

18.6 £

Confirmation of telephonic
order to Mr Brown today

UNION GROUP ENGINEERING.

INSPECTION ✗
DELIVERY Collect
TERMS Cash.

This was a landmark case which established Sydney Smith as one of the leading forensic pathologists in Britain. 'He was one of the few,' wrote Jürgen Thornald in his appreciation of Smith, 'who dared to challenge the Spilsbury legend.' He also demonstrated a refreshingly different approach in that he did not rely solely on his own skills and experience. As the investigation of Helen Priestly's death showed, he exercised great intuition but, at every turn, sought help and corroboration from other experts. This, of course, was not Spilsbury's way, but a tribute to Smith's approach came from the unlikely quarter of Jeannie Donald's defence counsel who described his work as, 'careful and meticulous preparation unparalleled in the history of this old court.' 'This old court' was the High Court at Edinburgh whence the trial had been moved to avoid any hint of local prejudice in Aberdeen. 'It was a change', said Smith dryly, 'greatly appreciated by the thrifty citizens of Aberdeen, since the expenses of the High Court would be met by the Crown, and not fall on the Aberdeen rates.' 'The Patriarch', as Smith's students liked to call him, was in the ascendancy.

While the Aberdeen child murder investigation was in progress, Smith received a letter from Lord Trenchard, Commissioner of the Metropolitan Police, asking for his advice about setting up a medico-legal laboratory for the police. The two men met in London and Trenchard, who described himself as 'an old man in a hurry', quickly drew up plans to start a laboratory at the Hendon Police College. Smith specified the equipment needed for the laboratories and buildings at the college were suitably adapted. In less than a year, the laboratory was in full operation.

Trenchard offered Smith the post of Director but he turned it down, making way for Dr James Davidson, a lecturer in his department at Edinburgh, to become the first Director. It was a considerable tribute to Smith that he was approached for his views on this innovative step in forensic investigation and he became a regular lecturer at Hendon.

Always a traveller, Smith decided to take his wife on a round-the-world trip in 1935, making a visit to Australia for professional reasons and to New Zealand to see family and friends. While in Sydney en route to Melbourne to attend a British Medical Association meeting, he became involved in what he described as 'one of the most extraordinary cases of my career'. This was the infamous Shark Arm affair. On 25 April, a startling phenomenon occurred in the Coogee Aquarium which housed a fourteen-foot shark caught by two local fishermen. When this captive denizen of the deep disgorged the contents of its stomach, spectators were horrified to see included a human arm severed at the shoulder. This grisly relic bore a distinctive tattoo of two boxers squaring up to each other which enabled the police to identify the individual to whom the arm belonged. In a list of missing persons were several men with tattoos and, by a process of elimination, the police confirmed that the owner of that particular boxing motif was one James Smith. The arm was identified by his wife and brother and further corroboration came from fingerprinting, for it appeared that Mr Smith was known to the police.

It seemed that James Smith had left home on 8 April, ostensibly to go on a fishing trip with another man whose identity he did not divulge to his wife. The question which the Australian authorities were keen to answer was whether the 'Shark Arm', as it was now called, had been ripped off by a shark, suggesting an accidental or possibly suicidal death, or dismembered by an act suggesting something more sinister. The fact that a visiting British Medical Association delegation of 157 doctors, including a distinguished forensic pathologist, was in the country, offered an ideal opportunity to secure an authoritative opinion.

Sydney Smith was asked to examine his namesake's arm although he admitted his expertise in bites lay more with the camel than the shark. Nevertheless, he had no doubt that the arm in question had been severed at the shoulder joint by a clean incision and that, after the head of the bone had been freed from its socket, the remaining tissues were cut away. The condition of the blood and tissues, despite the fact that the arm had been in the shark's stomach for at least a week, showed that the arm had been severed after death. There was every indication, therefore, of foul play.

No other portions of James Smith's body came to light but it was known that he had spent a holiday in a rented cottage on the coast at Cronulla with Patrick Brady, a forger known to the police. Brady denied any involvement in Smith's disappearance but implicated Reg Holmes, a Sydney boat builder, in forgery dealings. Brady was nevertheless charged with murdering Smith and three days later, following a sensational boat chase in Sydney Harbour, Holmes was apprehended. He had a bullet wound in the head, which was possibly self-inflicted, and he told the arresting officers that Brady had killed Smith and disposed of the body. Two weeks later, Reg Holmes, who would have been a star witness at Brady's trial, was shot dead in his car.

Sydney Smith's reconstruction of the crime, pieced together from police information, was that Brady and Smith quarrelled at Cronulla and Smith was killed. It was known that a tin trunk was missing from the cottage and it was supposed that the body was cut up and put into the trunk for disposal at sea. The problem was that the trunk was too small to accommodate every portion of the dismembered corpse. The piece left over was the left forearm, which by a stroke of fate was the only part of the body to bear any visible identification. The offending limb was roped to the side of the trunk and, during its burial at sea, was torn loose by a shark which nature determined should disgorge its stomach contents in a public aquarium. It was an extraordinary story and one which Sydney Smith acknowledged as a great deal stranger than fiction. Patrick Brady was tried for murder in September 1935 and acquitted. He denied the allegations right up to the time of his death in August 1965 and the mystery of the Shark Arm Case died with him.

While on board ship returning to Britain after his visit to the Antipodes, Sydney Smith learned the first details of a case in which he would be embroiled on reaching home. The remains of two women had been found in a gulley near Dumfriesshire on the Carlisle to Edinburgh road on 29 September 1935. These relics were taken to Smith's laboratory in Edinburgh where they were examined by his assistant, Dr W. Gilbert Millar, and Professor John Glaister of Glasgow University.

Apart from the grim nature of the discovery which eventually amounted to seventy pieces of two dismembered bodies, the case was significant for a number of other reasons. The perpetrator of these two murders and subsequent disposal by dissection was a doctor and the investigation which followed was distinguished by some remarkable forensic innovation. Sydney Smith and his department played a major role in this but chief credit went to John Glaister. The full story is therefore told in the next chapter which is devoted to Glaister's life and work. Suffice it to say here that Smith played a characteristically unselfish role from the moment he arrived back in Edinburgh on 7 November. He was consulted by the Chief Constables of Edinburgh and Lancaster to assist in identifying the remains. One of his university colleagues, Professor James Brash, Regius Professor of Anatomy, was already helping the police working alongside Glaister.

The trial of Dr Buck Ruxton took place at Manchester in March 1936. Sydney Smith was the last witness to give evidence and he was cross-examined by Norman Birkett who had so impressed him at the trial of Annie Hearn. Birkett was defending Ruxton and had been advised on the medical evidence by Sir Bernard Spilsbury. Smith made it clear that the two bodies had been dismembered after death by means of disarticulation at the joints, 'carried out in a sufficiently expert manner to show that the operator was quite familiar with human anatomy'.

The murderous Indian doctor from Lancaster was found guilty of killing his wife and maid and he went to the gallows on 12 May 1936. A curious footnote to this case was provided by the discovery among the scattered remains of Ruxton's victims of a Cyclopean eye. This is an unusual phenomenon in which the eyes of a malformed animal, usually a sheep or pig, fuse into one. Even more rarely, this malformation can occur in a human being. The condition takes its name from the one-eyed monster described by Homer in his *Odyssey* and named the Cyclops. In the Greek story, the monstrous Cyclops was blinded when Odysseus destroyed his single eye.

The Cyclopean eye which featured in the Ruxton case was of animal origin and had evidently been fixed at one time in preserving fluid. Smith's explanation was that Ruxton, who had an interest in ophthalmology, probably kept the eye as a preserved specimen. A possible explanation for the eye being found with the remains of his victims was that he emptied a jar of preservative over them and inadvertently tipped out the Cyclopean eye. Smith, in his memoirs, drew attention to a literary reference to the Cyclops made by Thomas de Quincey the essayist, in a piece entitled *A Vision of Sudden Death*, published in 1849. 'But what was Cyclops doing here?' he wrote. 'Had the medical man recommended northern air, or how?' He recollected, from such explanations as he volunteered, that he had an interest at stake in some suit-at-law pending in Lancaster; so that probably he had got himself transferred to this station for the purpose of connecting with his professional pursuits an instant readiness for the calls of the lawsuit'. This story, published in *Blackwood's Magazine* under the title *The English Mail Coach* was thick with coincidence, particularly bearing in mind Ruxton's residence at Lancaster.

Sydney Smith was at the peak of his career and had attained international status in the late 1930s when he was appointed as adviser to the World Health Organisation. He visited Ceylon in his advisory role to review the country's medico-legal services and to recommend improvements. It was a project in which he had something of a vested interest for the Professor of Forensic Medicine at Colombo University, Dr G.S.W. de Saram, was a former student. Not surprisingly, while in Ceylon, the visiting expert was prevailed upon to give his opinion of a controversial murder case going through the courts at the time.

As the decade drew to a close, so the Second World War loomed in the shadows. At the age of fifty-seven and with his particular talents, Smith was of greatest use for the war effort as a back-room boy. He spent the next five years investigating the ballistic characteristics of military ordnance and working for the War Office as a consultant in medico-legal matters. One of the factors he looked at was the penetrative power of various types of ammunition, finding, for example, that American cartridges produced more powerful effects than those manufactured in Britain. The chemical composition of the different propellants accounted for this discrepancy but the British manufacturers were not keen to give up their use of cordite.

The behaviour of high-velocity bullets was very much part of Smith's stock-in-trade and the war years allowed him to extend his already considerable knowledge of the subject. The home front produced its own casualties and, tragically, not always due to enemy action. One night in July 1940, a Royal Air Force Sergeant challenged a car being driven late at night in Edinburgh after an air-raid warning had sounded. The car, which did not stop, was being driven to police headquarters in the city and one of the passengers was the Assistant Chief Constable. The Sergeant fired at the car as it sped by and a .303 bullet passed through the celluloid rear-window, striking the Assistant Chief Constable in the face. The unfortunate officer died three days later and the RAF Sergeant was charged with assault and culpable homicide.

Although it was thought that only one shot had been fired, an examination of the car revealed a number of holes in the vehicle, including two in the windscreen, and there were dents in the metalwork. Consequently, it appeared as if at least two, and possibly more, shots had been fired. Smith carried out the post-mortem on the policeman and was able to reconstruct the course of the single deadly bullet which severely wounded him and caused his death. The bullet, a .303 aluminium-tipped projectile with a cupro-nickel jacket, struck the man on the right side of the jaw, completely shattering the bone and disintegrating as a result of the impact. Fragments of the bullet punched holes in the windscreen and the aluminium tip struck the metal frame and ricocheted to the back of the car where it was found on the rear seat.

Lord Aitchison, presiding judge at the High Court of Justiciary, ruled that although subject to military discipline, the RAF marksman was still within the law of the land. It appeared that he was legitimately armed in the post-Dunkirk period, with invasion fears running high when servicemen on leave took loaded weapons home. The Sergeant was on leave and had spent several hours that evening carousing with friends. When the air-raid siren sounded at about midnight, he took it on himself to act as a roadside sentry. Before the police car appeared, he challenged and threatened a car driven by an Auxiliary Fire Service officer. Then came the shooting tragedy. Despite his protestations that he was entitled to fire on vehicles not answering his challenge during an air raid, the RAF Sergeant was found guilty. He received a rather lenient sentence of six months' imprisonment.

In another tragedy on the home front, Smith was called in to examine a Home Guardsman shot dead during an exercise ostensibly involving blank ammunition. The exercise was staged near Edinburgh in the summer of 1942 and involved both regular troops and the Home Guard. The mock battle was stopped as soon as it was realised that one of the participants had been badly wounded. The man had been hit with a high-velocity .303 bullet which disintegrated on impact, creating injuries from which he later died.

Eyewitness accounts of the way the soldier reacted when struck by the bullet enabled Smith to determine the direction of the shot. Assisted by detectives from Edinburgh CID, he found an empty cartridge case that had fired a live round, among a number of blanks in an area occupied by a force of twenty-six soldiers representing an attacking group during the exercise. The rifles used by this group were collected by the police and test shots fired from each weapon.

Sydney Smith, a pioneering forensic ballistics expert, was in his element. He was able very quickly to identify the rifle which had fired the fatal shot by distinctive marks made on the cartridge case by the firing pin. The man responsible for this weapon had decided to make the military exercise more realistic by firing the occasional live round of ammunition. Following psychiatric examination he was found to have acted under a sense of diminished responsibility.

After the cessation of hostilities, Smith took part in a commission to assess the medical aspects of German war crimes. He and his colleagues, meeting in Frankfurt in 1946, heard a great deal of evidence about medical experiments carried out in the Nazi concentration camps. Every conceivable type of experiment was conducted, ranging from the pseudo-scientific to the merely sadistic. What struck the Allied doctors was that given access to unlimited human guinea pigs and with no ethical constraints, the experimenters worked without objectives or proper methods. 'The experiments,' wrote Smith, 'were not merely carried out with gross indifference to the value of human life and callous disregard to human suffering, but were incompetent in both conception and execution from a purely scientific point of view.'

In December of the following year, the world of forensic medicine mourned the loss of Sir Bernard Spilsbury. The circumstances of his suicide were tragic but a hint of rancour came through in Sydney Smith's appraisal of the man; after all, they had endured several bitter clashes. He referred to his rival's death as, 'the inquest on his last case of suicide – and there was no room for doubt this time – he was the deceased.' Although he sincerely mourned his colleague, Smith felt there was really no place for the stubbornness of opinion that was Spilsbury's hallmark. 'One might almost hope that there will never be another Bernard Spilsbury,' he wrote in his autobiography. If it was a wish, it was one which came true, for the up-and-coming medical detectives were men of a different breed and there was not to be another Spilsbury among them.

Smith himself reached the pinnacle of his career in 1949 when he was knighted for his services to forensic medicine and, as the 1950s dawned, he was planning for retirement. His opposite number in the Chair of Forensic Medicine at Glasgow University, John Glaister, was well established and building his own considerable reputation. The two men had worked together on a number of cases and, in 1931, collaborated in the writing of a book on *Recent Advances in Forensic Medicine*. It was typical of Smith's attitude to break away from Spilsbury's tendency towards isolationism and to use his knowledge to help others.

In London, Spilsbury's old territory, Francis Camps and Keith Simpson were making their mark. Simpson had published his textbook, *Forensic Medicine*, in 1947, as if to put up a marker in the year of Spilsbury's death. Although this book seriously challenged Smith's own contribution to learning on the subject, he was generous in his acknowledgement of the newcomer. Indeed, in due course, Smith handed on to Simpson the editorship of *Taylor's Principles and Practice of Medical Jurisprudence*, which he had managed so masterfully for thirty years. Simpson would say of The Patriarch in due course, 'He was like a second father to me as I grew up in the field of forensic medicine.'

It was part of Smith's natural gifts as a teacher to encourage the next generation of forensic practitioners and he did so with characteristic generosity. In return, they sought to honour him by seeking his advice in their new enterprises. In the late 1940s, Simpson and Camps led a small group which proposed to establish a British Association in Forensic Medicine. Their idea was to provide a forum wherein forensic specialists could exchange experiences and learn from each other. As Simpson described it in his autobiography, they met at the 'Bon Accord' restaurant in Soho and invited 'the only man who at that time stood head and shoulders above everyone in both academic stature and experience' to be the first President of the Association. Sir Sydney Smith accepted graciously: the era of the lone expert, personified by the late Bernard Spilsbury, was ended.

Meanwhile, Smith began a trend which his successors would follow in due course; this was to use his expertise internationally to help solve important cases in countries lacking forensic capability. He travelled a great deal during the early 1950s before he retired, visiting New Zealand, the land of his birth, and also Egypt, which had been a kind of promised land for him in his younger days. 1952 was a momentous year, filled with academic engagements and medico–legal casework. He advised on a murder case in Kenya, lectured in Canada and undertook further work for the World Health Organisation.

Despite this busy programme, he found time to fly out to Ceylon to assist his friend and former student, Dr de Saram, who was involved in a difficult murder case in which his professional judgement was severely questioned. 'The facts of the case were simple,' wrote Smith years later. Mrs Sathasiran, estranged wife of the former captain of Ceylon's cricket team, was found dead in the garage of her home in Colombo. Dr de Saram was called and he examined the body about an hour after it was discovered and carried out a full post-mortem on the following day. In the meantime, Sathasiran was arrested and charged with murdering his wife. Ten days after the crime, the Sathasirans' servant, William, confessed that he had helped his master commit the murder by subduing the victim's struggles when she was strangled. A key factor in his confession was that William said all this occurred before 9 a.m. and that, by 9.30 he had sold the jewellery stripped from the body and given to him in payment for his services. This statement was corroborated by the jeweller who had bought the articles.

Dr de Saram's examination of the victim led him to different conclusions about the likely time of her death. The extent of rigor mortis in the body indicated that death had occurred between 10 a.m. and noon. It was known that Mrs Sathasiran had eaten breakfast comprising a type of pasta, grated coconut and milk around 8.15 a.m. The state of digestion of this meal as seen in her stomach and intestines, made it apparent that she had eaten breakfast some three hours before meeting her death. This conclusion was broadly confirmed by the temperature of the body. Despite the bland assurances to the contrary conveyed in detective fiction, it is extremely difficult to establish the time of death from the condition of the body, and rarely possible to do so with precision. Taking all factors into account, Dr de Saram's estimate of the likely time of death was between 10 and 11.30 a.m. which was at variance with William's confession.

At a preliminary magistrates inquiry, William was pardoned and he agreed to stand as a witness for the Crown against his former master. Sathasiran was sent for trial, charged with murdering his wife before 9.30 on the morning of 9 October 1951. The specific reference to time of death cast a shadow over Dr de Saram's professional judgement and the prosecution did everything it could to discredit his opinion.

After he had read all the evidence, Smith reconstructed the crime in his laboratory at Edinburgh with the help of defence counsel who had travelled from Ceylon to seek his opinion. He believed the facts showed that after Sathasiran left the house by taxi at 10.35 a.m., an event which was well corroborated, his wife, only scantily dressed, went down into the kitchen where she encountered William. Aged eighteen and only in her employ for a week, William became sexually excited and attempted to assault Mrs Sathasiran. When she resisted, he seized her by the neck, throttling her into unconsciousness, as a result of which she urinated, leaving a tell-tale stain on her petticoat. Smith's experienced eye had spotted that the extent of the stain was more in keeping with the victim being in a standing rather than a prone position.

As a result of this initial attack, the victim sagged against the doorway, bruising her back and tearing her sari. She had sustained a bruise between the shoulder blades and there were tears in her clothing. Smith told the defence lawyers to confirm whether or not there was a projection of any kind about three and a half feet from the floor, on or near, the kitchen door. His belief was that the murder resulted unintentionally from a sexually motivated assault.

By the time the case came to trial, Sir Sydney Smith was already in his final year's programme at Edinburgh University. Nevertheless, he flew to Ceylon on 20 May 1952 in order to appear in court on behalf of the defence. One of his first actions was to visit the scene of the crime. On the wall between the kitchen and the garage he found a staple which substantiated his view of how the victim's back was bruised. The jeweller's evidence supporting William's statement about the time he sold the murder victim's rings and necklace was proved to be perjured. Consequently, the trial progressed chiefly on the testimony of medical experts. Dr de Saram's reputation took a knock when the Solicitor-General obtained the judge's agreement to question him as a hostile witness. Moreover, the doctor faced the massed ranks of the prosecution's experts, representing every conceivable discipline including a Professor of Mathematics.

But de Saram had Sydney Smith in his corner and, as usual, his preparation had been meticulous. He had given instructions for experiments to be carried out on body cooling and the corpses of three executed murderers were obtained for the purpose. Dressed in clothing similar to that worn by Mrs Sathasiran and placed in conditions simulating those of the murder scene, their temperatures were taken every half hour. The results showed that the bodies lost 5.2 degrees of heat in seven hours. This compared with the murder victim's loss of 5.2 degrees over ten hours if the prosecution's estimate of time of death was correct. Smith's contention, supported by his experiments, was that Mrs Sathasiran died several hours after 9 a.m. which was the time given by William in his confession. This was born out by independent witnesses who claimed to have seen the murder victim and to have spoken to her on the telephone after 10.30 a.m.

Faced with this powerful rebuttal of its evidence, the prosecution presented a mass of information drawn from learned textbooks to bolster their argument. Hoping to wound him, Crown counsel asked Smith why he was prepared to support Dr de Saram in this case while he had refused to accept the evidence of a much more distinguished person, Sir Bernard Spilsbury, in the Fox case. Of course, the two cases could not be compared and, in any event, the role of the forensic expert was to speak with experience supported by fact which Smith had done so admirably. The jury thought so too and brought in a unanimous verdict of 'Not Guilty'. Feeling elated but tired, Sydney Smith flew back to Britain on 30 May. Turning over in his mind the events of the previous few days, he noted for later inclusion in his autobiography, 'I had quite forgotten the Fox case until it was mentioned to me at the trial.'

His confrontation with Spilsbury had, after all, occurred over twenty years before and, now, approaching his seventieth year, he was shortly to retire. He attended the Coronation of Queen Elizabeth II at Westminster Abbey on 2 June 1953 and recounted an amusing incident which occurred afterwards. Unable to find a taxi to return him from the abbey to his hotel, he walked, attired in his university robes, through the crowds of Piccadilly. His scarlet gown and black velvet berette caused some excitement and drew the remark, 'here comes a bloody bishop', from a bystander.

Sir Sydney retired from Edinburgh's Chair of Forensic Medicine in 1953 and, with the praise of his colleagues and students ringing in his ears, set off with his wife to Lebanon and Ceylon on behalf of the World Health Organisation. While he was relieved of the burden of teaching, his retirement was really only a matter of administrative nomenclature. After nine months abroad, he returned to Britain and was honoured at Edinburgh by being presented with his portrait painted by Sir William Hutchinson, President of the Royal Scottish Academy. It was a fitting tribute to a man whose association with the university spanned half a century. In 1954 he was elected Rector of the University, an honour which he deeply appreciated.

While in Montreal in August 1954 on a world tour, he suffered a minor heart attack and was ordered to rest for a few weeks. He had already agreed to assist in an arsenic poisoning case in New Zealand and, despite the setback in his health, confirmed that he would give evidence for the defence at the re-trial of James Wilson due to start in Auckland in October. Wilson had been tried earlier but the jury could not agree on a verdict.

There was no greater authority on arsenic poisoning than Sydney Smith and from his review of the medical evidence in this case, he did not believe Wilson poisoned his wife. When he gave evidence he was asked what his experience was in regard to arsenical poisoning. He mentioned his time in Egypt and answered in a matter-of-fact way, 'I don't suppose I saw more than one a week.' This was a nonchalant way of saying more than 500! He was the only witness called by the defence and his calm authority won Wilson an acquittal. Mrs Wilson's death remained a mystery but it was known that she was devoted to self medication. Analysis of her hair and nails showed that she had ingested small doses of arsenic over several months. It was thought that she might have dosed herself with arsenic as a treatment for a skin rash. The only book in the house was a well-thumbed copy of *Domestic Medical Practice* which contained a reference to an arsenical preparation for skin rashes.

The Smiths continued their world tour, visiting Australia and Ceylon, and spending three months in Egypt, before finally returning to Britain in 1956. Political aggravation fuelled by fierce nationalism was brewing under President Nasser and the world's attention was drawn to the future of the Suez Canal. The tense atmosphere was reminiscent of their first time in Egypt nearly forty years before but they were greeted with friendly Egyptian hospitality everywhere they went and left the country before the hostilities over Suez began.

Smith acknowledged that while murder was of great interest to the public, it was only of minor significance so far as general crime was concerned. In more than thirty years of specialised practice in forensic medicine, he had seen many great advances in scientific methods – indeed he had pioneered some himself. He acknowledged that his professional career had provided him with great interest but low remuneration. Recalling a case in which his opinion had been instrumental in securing a not guilty verdict for a man charged with murder, he recorded the discussion which resulted over payment. The accused man's solicitors wrote to him asking him to state his fee. His suggestion that one hundred guineas would be appropriate prompted a letter pointing out that medical and scientific specialists usually only charged about ten guineas. Smith returned their letter having written on it the question, 'What is your client's life worth?' He received his cheque the next day.

The last case in which Sydney Smith took an active part was one that called on an area of specialised knowledge with which he had become acquainted during his time in Egypt. The Welsh Mummy case, as it was termed by the newspapers, caused headlines in 1960 when the mummified body of a woman in her sixties was found in the cupboard of a house at Rhyl in North Wales. The body was identified as the remains of Mrs Frances Knight, a semi-invalid who had been a lodger in Mrs Sarah Jane Harvey's terrace house in the seaside town.

The body had been discovered by Mrs Harvey's son, who was painting the interior of the house. He opened a cupboard on the landing which, from the time of his childhood, had always been kept mysteriously locked. Among all the cobwebs and dirt, he saw a human foot protruding from a mound of clothing on the floor. The police were called and Dr Gerald Evans, the pathologist, found a human body, the shrunken flesh of which he described as being hard as a statue. As it emerged later, the body had been holed up in the cupboard of Mrs Harvey's house for twenty years.

Sarah Harvey told the police that Mrs Knight was very frail when she came to board with her. She suffered from rheumatism which affected her mobility and caused her a great deal of pain. She found her lodger one night on the floor of her room – 'I am in an awful lot of pain and would rather be dead', she was claimed to have said. Later, when Mrs Harvey called in on her, she found her dead. The landlady's reaction was to drag the body out to the landing and put it into the cupboard. She hung up a few fly papers and wrapped an eiderdown around the corpse. When she locked the cupboard, she had effectively entombed Mrs Knight's remains for twenty years. So firmly rooted was the body to the floor of the cupboard that a garden spade had to be used to prise it free.

Apart from a number of discrepancies in Sarah Harvey's story, and a few obvious questions such as, why did she not report the death of an ailing lodger to the authorities, there was the awkward discovery of what appeared to be a ligature around the dead woman's neck. It looked like murder, and sixty-five-year-old Mrs Harvey was charged with its commission.

Dr Francis Camps was called in by the defence after Sarah Harvey had been committed for trial at the Assize Court in Ruthin, Denbighshire. He enlisted the help of Sir Sydney Smith who, apart from his wide experience as a pathologist, probably knew more than anyone at the time about the medical aspects of mummification. This condition is unusual in Britain but is by no means rare. Indeed Camps caused quite a stir when he said that he probably encountered some four mummies a year.

Sarah Harvey's landing cupboard, the doors of which permitted air to pass through, provided ideal conditions to induce mummification in the body of a frail, emaciated woman. Dr Evans's scientific work on the body and his pathological report were highly praised. He described a piece of 'coiled string-like material' found on the left-hand side of the neck in which there was a groove. The prosecution case was that Mrs Knight had been strangled with a stocking by Sarah Harvey for the purpose of acquiring her lodger's £2 per week alimony.

Mrs Harvey had shown herself to be something of a schemer and had indeed regularly collected Mrs Knight's alimony after she was dead.

The defence believed that Mrs Knight died of natural causes, probably from disseminated sclerosis, and that the groove in her neck was no more than a post-mortem change and was not due to a homicidal ligature. Smith and Camps believed that the significance of the stocking lay less in its indications of murder than in the old wives' remedy of wrapping a sock or stocking around the neck at bedtime to cure a chesty cold. They believed that, following death, Mrs Knight's body underwent putrefaction in the normal way which included the decomposition of fly eggs and destruction of the soft tissues by maggots. As the skin overall dried slowly, that under the stocking was kept moist with decomposition products, causing the neck to swell. Under those conditions the loosely tied stocking caused a groove or depression to form around the neck. Sir Sydney was able to support this interpretation from his experience and to provide photographic evidence.

Dr Evans's conclusion that it was not possible to ascertain the cause of Mrs Knight's death together with the known view of the defence experts that there was an innocent explanation for the stocking around the neck, brought the trial to an end on the fifth day. Perhaps the presence in court of so eminent a witness as Sydney Smith persuaded the prosecution that they were not on firm ground. Mrs Harvey was, consequently, found not guilty of murder but was convicted of falsely obtaining money, ostensibly for Mrs Knight, by pretending that she was still alive. She perpetuated this fraud from May 1940 until April 1960, a foolishness for which she was sentenced to fifteen months' imprisonment.

Sydney Smith retired in 1953, relinquishing his chair as Regius Professor, a post he had held for twenty-five years. He was appointed Emeritus Professor and Rector of the University. Glowing with the warmth of the tributes paid them by the University, he and his wife, Kitty, set off for a long visit to New Zealand. They returned to Edinburgh in 1955 and were welcomed with a dinner and reception provided by the Students' Council. To be honoured by his students was as important to him as the accolades received from academic colleagues. Keith Simpson, in a generous appreciation of Smith, wrote, 'His sage advice was sought by young aspirants the world over ....'.

In 1959, Sir Sydney published his memoirs in a book entitled *Mostly Murder* which he dedicated to Kitty, 'a good companion for half a century'. Lord Cameron, in his preface, remarked on Smith's journey through life which had been, 'full of interest, crowned with honour and the love of friends'. The author himself was more matter-of-fact; informing his readers that his book was, 'a plain, unvarnished tale without embellishment or emotion'. He hoped that readers would find in it '... something of interest in another man's work'. From the man who had edited *Taylor's Principles and Practice of Medical Jurisprudence* for thirty years, this was indeed a modest ambition.

Smith's 'good companion', Kitty, died in 1960 and he soldiered on, continuing to publish new editions of *Mostly Murder*. When he died in 1969, it was remarked that he would be remembered for his writing as much as any of his achievements. He was known affectionately as 'The Patriarch', respected head of the family of forensic pathologists. In the first edition of his book, *Forensic Medicine*, published in 1925, he wrote, 'A knowledge of medicine and a stock of common sense are not in themselves sufficient.' He emphasised that the medical jurist must have special knowledge. This was not mere preaching but an ideal which he practised throughout his career. His willingness to embrace new methods and to combine his knowledge with that of others to ensure the best possible outcome, were the hallmarks of a professional career which spanned half a century.

Smith's signal contribution to his profession was acknowledged in numerous tributes after his death. Francis Camps, describing him as, 'A burly, cheerful man', spoke of his charm and natural abilities as an 'academic politician'. These were gifts admired by his peers in a profession not particularly noted for its generosity of spirit. Further editions of *Mostly Murder* continued to appear after Sir Sydney's death and the 1982 edition was reviewed in the *Medical News Guide* published in Bombay. 'This book should be read by everyone who has something to do with forensic medicine,' wrote the reviewer. There was perhaps no finer tribute to a man whose forensic genius had made him an internationally respected figure.

Chapter Three

THE PROFESSOR

John Glaister

AS A YOUNG MAN John Glaister had a leaning towards light entertainment and thought briefly about a career on the stage. While he possessed a natural talent for impersonation or what he liked to call mimicry, the weight of history and family tradition was against him. His father, Dr John Glaister, 'Old John', as he would be called to differentiate him from his progeny of the same name, was a Glasgow general practitioner, destined to become Professor of Forensic Medicine at the city's university.

'Young John' was born in May 1892, the final addition to the Glaisters' family of two boys and four girls. His boyhood memories were of a Victorian father who he described as, 'both a popular and kenspeckle figure', the latter being a Scots word meaning 'conspicuous' and perhaps translated into the modern idiom as 'high profile'. With his duties as a busy medical practitioner, making his calls in style using a horse-drawn carriage, and lecturing on public health and other matters at St Mungo's College, 'Old John' often did not see his children for days on end.

The family lived in a large house attended by servants. The children were driven to school by the coachman and, in due course, the youngest Glaister found himself at Glasgow High School and compelled to learn Latin which, in common with most of his contemporaries, he loathed. Some of his strongest boyhood memories were of long columns of soldiers waiting patiently at Glasgow docks to board troopships bound for South Africa and the Boer War.

At the turn of the century, 'Old John' was appointed to the Regius Chair of Forensic Medicine at Glasgow University. The new position meant a change of address and the Glaister family moved into a large house in Woodside Place. University life entailed more regular working hours and his children saw more of their father. There were still unsocial hours to be worked though and when a medical report was required 'Old John' clattered away on his typewriter until late at night. He spurned the idea of taking on a secretary with the same force that he rejected the installation of a telephone. When the family were enjoying the pleasures of their country house in Dumfriesshire, a telegraph boy had to be despatched from nearby Thornhill with a message summoning the professor if his forensic skills were needed urgently at some crime scene.

In his autobiography, 'Young John' recalled the moment he was called to his father's study to give an account of his progress at school. He knew his reports told a depressing story and his father advocated greater concentration. When asked what he intended to do when he left school, the seventeen-year-old lad ventured to suggest that he might go to London to study at the Academy of Dramatic Art. 'Forget it', was his father's unequivocal reply. He advised a university course, suggesting first medicine and then the law. Father and son agreed that the best way to dispel the poor school results was to employ a private tutor. William Love prepared John Glaister for entry at Glasgow University within a few months and the pupil later paid his tutor a generous compliment when he said, 'he taught me to learn how to learn'.

His years as a medical student merged with the onset of the First World War. They were enjoyable years after he had surmounted the curiosity of his fellow undergraduates who were bemused by the prospects of 'Young John' being lectured to by 'Old John'. When they realised that he was treated in exactly the same way as themselves, their curiosity was satisfied. Glaister had his share of memorable experiences as every prospective doctor does and he recalled a number of them in his memoirs. There were some amusing interludes and none more so than working among the poor who lived in Glasgow's slum tenements. He was called out one night with a fellow student to attend an expectant mother and was guided by a lighted candle to the woman's bedside in a dingy, one-roomed apartment. While they looked after their patient, they also had to contend with marauding bed bugs which crept over the bedding and dropped from the ceiling. Their attention was as much taken up by keeping the blood-sucking bugs at bay as it was looking after the patient and new uses were found for the ether which they carried in their medical bags – *Cimex lectularius* proved vulnerable to its anaesthetic powers.

Like most young men of his generation, when the war came Glaister wanted to join up immediately. His family and university teachers prevailed on him to finish his studies and he reluctantly deferred to their wishes. Nevertheless, he and a fellow student volunteered their services to help at the military hospital which was set up at Glasgow's Hyde Park Locomotive Works. He helped to treat many of the war's lesser casualties – soldiers with trench foot and heart disorders. 'Young John' passed his final examinations in March 1916 and, within weeks, had been commissioned as a doctor in the Royal Army Medical Corps.

After a couple of home postings he was informed that he was to be sent to Egypt. He said hurried farewells to his parents and to his fiancée, Isobel, known to all her intimates as 'Muff', before setting out on an overland route to Alexandria via Taranto in Italy. Captain Glaister was posted to Gaza as a regimental medical officer, where he joined a field ambulance unit with little to do but kill time by playing gramophone records and debating the reason for their posting. The purpose became all too apparent one evening when a soldier reported sighting an approaching camel train. 'We rushed out,' said Glaister, 'and the entire stretch of skyline seemed filled by the length of the plodding convoy coming towards us.'

There were a hundred or more camels each carrying two wounded soldiers slung in nets on their backs. 'It was a sight', wrote Glaister, 'to make even the most hardened medical orderly wince.' The men were Turkish prisoners, many of them seriously wounded at Beersheba and kept confined for days in caves before being sent by convoy to receive medical treatment. The doctors and medical orderlies worked long into the night dealing with badly infected wounds necessitating an endless series of amputations. Once the surgery was completed, it became apparent that typhus was rampant among the survivors. The fever was spread by the lice with which the men were infested and strict hygiene was enforced within an isolation area patrolled by armed guards. It was a nightmarish episode, and when it was finished, only eleven out of the original 200 casualties survived.

This would have been a harrowing experience for any young man but doubly depressing for one who was a newly qualified doctor. 'All I wanted,' wrote Glaister, 'was to be given the home leave due to me.' He returned to Scotland and he and Muff were married in Glasgow Cathedral on 25 May 1918. In due course, he was again posted to the Middle East to serve in a military hospital at Ludd in Egypt. One of his first tasks was to set up an emergency unit to deal with an outbreak of bacillary dysentery among Turkish prisoners. He contracted the disease himself and was reduced to a low ebb, losing a great deal of weight and picking up influenza while in the base hospital in Cairo. He was sent home on a hospital ship eventually arriving in a poor condition at University College Hospital, Birmingham, where he was meant to convalesce. One of the doctors there was a friend of his father's and he pulled a few strings to allow 'Young John' to go home to Glasgow. 'When I did reach home,' he wrote later, 'I was still skeleton thin and anaemic, so that my young bride walked past me on the station platform.'

When he was finally demobilised in August 1919, 'Young John' settled down to the life of a married man and contemplated the direction of his future career. He knew that he was destined to take up medico-legal work and had already obtained a post as part-time lecturer at Glasgow University. But, first, he would gain experience in general practice. He and Muff moved into rented accommodation in the city's North Kelvinside district and he 'put up his plate'. After a slow start, he acquired some 300 patients on his panel and began to acquire work from the Ministry of Pensions. He also started to build up the medico-legal side of his portfolio, working, as he liked to describe it, as 'a back-room boy' in his father's forensic team.

It was not long before he decided to give up general practice and devote his attention to medical jurisprudence. Things had been progressing sufficiently well to allow the couple to move with their two young daughters to a house in Fitzroy Place. When 'Young John' was appointed lecturer in medical jurisprudence by the City of Glasgow Police, his future direction seemed assured. But he had set himself a severe schedule, carrying out research leading to a doctorate of medicine and also studying to become a barrister. For good measure, he was also planning a thesis which he hoped would earn him a doctorate of science.

The laboratory aspects of forensic work had captured his interest and it was in the realms of the 'backroom' that he first made his mark. In 1901, a young German military doctor, Paul Uhlenhuth, working in the University of Greifswald, announced that he had found a way of differentiating between human and animal blood. Researchers had long been seeking a way of overcoming this barrier to crime investigation and Uhlenhuth's precipitin test promised to be that breakthrough. What Glaister proposed to do was to eliminate doubt from the testing procedure due to incidental factors like temperature, the age of the bloodstain and the biological sera used in the test. He believed that only by putting the reliability of the precipitin test beyond doubt would British courts accept it as satisfactory. Here was the work of the true professional. Uhlenhuth had achieved the glory and all Glaister wanted was to turn the discovery into a reliable tool for the forensic investigator.

His other chosen field of backroom laboratory work was one in which he rightly received plaudits in due course as an innovator. This was his classification of mammalian hair, a task which had a Holmesian ring to it and one which represented another landmark for forensic investigators. Hairs were often found at a crime scene and the problem was to identify them as of human or animal origin in order to eliminate fruitless lines of investigation. Glaister wanted to create a standard reference table so that the origin of any hair sample could be identified. This work involved collecting reference samples from all manner of sources, including zoos, museums and taxidermists, and the task took several years to complete.

Both of his major pieces of research involved the minutiae of crime investigation. Forensic pioneers such as Dr Edmond Locard at the University of Lyon had shown the potential for solving crimes by examining trace evidence at the crime scene on both victim and suspect. The fact that even the slightest contact results in a transfer of such mundane materials as distinctive hairs and fibres, while violent contact may involve biological traces such as blood, saliva or semen, opened up a whole vista for forensic scientists. The methods for examining trace evidence have grown ever more sophisticated with the use of advanced chemical analysis. When Glaister was telling his students about the 'key of interchange', as he called the concept of trace evidence, he might have dreamed of identifying body fluids as unerringly as fingerprints. But it was to take well over half a century before the first murder conviction would be secured by means of genetic fingerprinting.

Glaister, father and son, frequently answered calls from the police together. 'Young John' had a happy apprenticeship and readily deferred to his father's experience. But, all the while, he was building up his own expertise and, in the year that he helped his father on the Merrett case, he was awarded his doctorate of medicine and was also called to the Bar at the Inner Temple. His work on the precipitin test was to have slightly ironic consequences for the father and son relationship when they both appeared as prosecution witnesses in a case tried at Edinburgh's High Court of Justiciary. The defence challenged the reliability of blood tests and asked 'Old John' why he had been so critical of them in a textbook he had written. Glaister senior answered that he had changed his views in light of recent advances and said that future references in his textbook would be amended. 'Young John' was unaware of this when his turn came to give evidence. As the author of the new research in blood testing, he was closely questioned by the defence. He was astute enough to realise that counsel was leading him on to say that he was an expert in this particular field, with the implication that Glaister senior knew little about these new advances and was merely relying on his son's knowledge. Sensing the trap, 'Young John' replied by saying that, although he carried out all the tests, the results were checked and corroborated by his father.

The Merrett case, tried in Edinburgh in 1927, brought together both the established and the emerging forensic talent of the time. The Glasgow team comprised Professor John Glaister and his son, who would be his successor in due course, and the Edinburgh pair were Professor Harvey Littlejohn and Sydney Smith, his eventual successor. Sir Bernard Spilsbury, of course, was one of the major participants and the full story has been told in Chapter One. The Glaisters' interpretation of the evidence, favouring murder rather than suicide, was shown by subsequent events to have been the more correct, although it was not accepted as such at the time.

Later that year, 'Young John' completed his thesis on mammalian hair and he was awarded a doctorate of science. He thus completed an intensive period of study which set him up as a highly qualified forensic practitioner and one thing was sure – there would be no shortage of opportunities to exercise his skills. Such an opportunity occurred in 1928 when, following Harvey Littlejohn's death,

Sydney Smith succeeded him in the chair at Edinburgh. This left a vacancy in Egypt when Smith gave up his eleven-year tenure of office and 'Young John' was invited to apply for the Chair of Forensic Medicine at the University of Cairo. Smith told him he would see almost as many medico-legal cases in a week in Egypt as he would see in an average year in Britain. Glaister was attracted by the proposition, not least because he believed that forensic medicine should be put on an international footing. In November 1928, John Glaister, with his wife and two daughters, sailed from Liverpool for Port Said.

With an average of 150 post-mortem examinations a month, the new professor soon realised the correctness of Sydney Smith's prediction. 'Shooting and stabbing were two favourite methods of murder in Cairo,' he wrote, and, 'There was nothing unusual in finding half a dozen overnight murders requiring attention when I arrived for work after breakfast'. Egypt's ancient traditions enabled him to write a footnote in the medical textbooks regarding the precipitin test. Professor Douglas Derry, Head of the Anatomy Department and a keen Egyptologist, invited John Glaister to accompany him on a number of 'digs'. The opportunity arose to be present at the unwrapping of a mummy from the Twelfth Dynasty. He took tissue samples from various organs and subjected them to the precipitin test, achieving positive results with material dating back between 3 and 4,000 years. The point was made that the test was reliable even when used on very old samples.

Access to ancient mummified material also enabled him to obtain perfectly preserved samples of hair to add to his already large collection. Indeed, his work on the subject had by now been set out in book form, comprising an atlas of 1,200 micro-photographs, with a very long title. *A Study of Hairs and Wools Belonging to the Mammalian Group of Animals, including a Special Study of Human Hair, Considered from the Medico-Legal Aspect*, was published in Cairo in 1931. The expense of printing the book was undertaken by the Egyptian Government and the author gratefully dedicated the work to King Fuad. Like his predecessor, Sydney Smith, he was invited to meet the King at the Abdine Palace which he found richly carpeted and full of pomp. The necessity for their father to wear court dress and a tarboosh on such occasions inevitably reduced the Glaister children to a state of girlish giggles.

Like his fellow forensic practitioners, John Glaister found that crime seemed to follow him even while on holiday. He and his wife were in Cyprus in 1928 when an important case came to trial involving two doctors accused of performing an abortion. As soon as Glaister's presence on the island was known, he was asked to help prepare the case for the Crown. A twenty-four-year-old Cypriot woman had died following an alleged attempt to induce an abortion. She had been treated in a clinic in Nicosia where she died following surgery which had resulted in a perforation of the uterus and caused a haemorrhage. Twelve hours later, without explanation, a man delivered the young woman's body wrapped in a sheet to her parents' home. Her history was that she had been having problems with menstruation and doctors prescribed tonic medicine and internal syringing. No suggestion was made that she might be pregnant, but her mother was advised that an operation was needed to scrape the uterus. It was this operation, poorly carried out, which had resulted in the woman's death. The post-mortem examination indicated that she was pregnant and that the surgical procedure performed by two doctors at the clinic amounted to an attempted abortion. The jury also took this view with the result that one doctor was found guilty of manslaughter while charges against the second doctor were dropped on grounds of insufficient evidence.

It was while on holiday in Cyprus the following year that John Glaister took another decisive step in his career. 'Old John' had written to tell him that he had decided to retire after thirty-three years in the professorial chair at Glasgow. There was thus an opportunity for the son to apply for the vacancy created by the father's departure, although he realised it was a hard act to follow. He acknowledged that 'Old John' was, in all respects, a living legend, yet the challenge was there and he was eminently qualified to succeed. He applied for the Regius Chair of Forensic Medicine to the Secretary of State for Scotland and awaited developments. Asked if he would be willing to attend for interview, he replied that he would let his application speak for him.

During the last weeks of their holiday in the Troodos Mountains in Cyprus in September 1931, John Glaister received a cable informing him that he had been appointed to the chair. 'Young John' had come of age and was now truly his own man. There were regrets at leaving Egypt but, from a professional point of view, he found the climate too deferential. While many men would have been flattered to command such admiration, John Glaister found it uncomfortable; 'Every man now and again needs to be told he is talking nonsense – even if only to give him the chance to prove himself correct,' he wrote later. So, after three years in the land of the Pharaohs, the Glaisters said their farewells and left to return to Scotland. Egypt had been but a brief interlude although, as events turned out, the connection had not been broken.

John Glaister was aware of the sort of remarks his succession to his father's position might provoke. But in truth, his professional credentials and reputation were beyond criticism and he had firm ideas about the future direction of forensic medicine. Certainly 'Old John' did not linger at the university to offer advice or, worse still, to interfere, '. . . he left the building and never returned to it,' said his son. Glaister realised that he would inevitably face opposition from the Old Guard, those who had been in practice while he was still a student, but he resolved to plot a course that would further both the independence and international outlook of his professional calling.

There was an early clash when he was privately taken to task by a Procurator Fiscal on account of his practice of sometimes appearing as a witness for the prosecution and, on others, for the defence. The Procurator told Glaister he objected to him giving evidence against the Crown doctors and ordered him not to do so again, threatening that he would not be asked to appear for the Crown in future. John Glaister was horrified at what he had been told and he invited the Procurator to repeat his instructions in the presence of witnesses. This was greeted with a sullen silence and the professor left, marking his disgust by slamming the door.

After just a few months in his new post John Glaister was asked by the University Principal if he would be willing to return to Egypt to lecture for a three-month period every year. The Egyptian Government had written to the university making this special request and it was agreed that he could be released during the non-teaching term. The Glaisters' return to Egypt was a pleasant experience, marred only by bad news from home. Muff had to return to England to see her brother who was dangerously ill, leaving John to see out the rest of the tour on his own. While at sea on board the *Orontes* bound for England in 1931, he received a cable informing him that both his father and mother had died. They succumbed at home within hours of each other from a virulent influenza epidemic which was raging in Britain. 'Old John's' passing and a sense of a chapter closing persuaded John Glaister to give up his arrangement with the Egyptian Government and despite attempts to dissuade him he stuck to his decision.

He threw himself whole-heartedly into his work at the university using his experience and quiet authority to guide a generation of students whose professional calling would one day take them into the witness box. It was a lonely place, he told them, and one where any hint of posing would be seen for what it was. 'I've always tried to be as natural as possible when giving evidence,' he wrote, in the belief that professional stature and a thorough knowledge of the subject were the chief requirements. He extolled the virtues of being concise, a habit he had picked up from 'Old John' whose answers to the probing questions of counsel frequently consisted of a string of affirmatives and negatives. He believed that the witness who sought to expand on his answers was a boon to opposing counsel; as the maxim had it, 'A witness in saying more than he ought frequently says more than he means'. Above all, he believed in the powers of accurate and close observation. A sensible working philosophy for the forensic expert was that things are not always what they seem.

In 1935, John Glaister's approach to forensic medicine was put to the test in a sensational murder case involving a member of his own profession whose criminal activities spilled over into Scotland. The story began on 29 September when a young Edinburgh woman visiting Dumfriesshire crossed a bridge on the

Edinburgh–Carlisle road. Glancing down into the stream running in a ravine beneath the bridge she saw what she thought was a human arm protruding from some sort of wrapping material. Susan Johnson returned to her hotel at Moffat and told her brother what she had seen. Alfred Johnson went to the spot and made a closer inspection; he discovered various human remains wrapped in newspapers and pieces of clothing. He called the police.

When the area was searched by officers of the Dumfriesshire Constabulary, four bundles were recovered, each containing portions of a human body together with other pieces strewn about the ravine. One bundle wrapped in a blouse contained two upper arms and four pieces of flesh; another consisted of a pillowcase, the grisly contents of which included two upper arm bones, two thigh bones, two lower leg bones and nine pieces of flesh. A third parcel wrapped in a piece of sheet enclosed seventeen pieces of flesh, and a fourth contained part of a trunk and the lower parts of two legs including the feet. There were also two heads, one of which was wrapped in a pair of child's rompers. These were the immediate discoveries but, as the police extended their searches, further portions of bodies were retrieved. Nearly a month later, a foot was found at a point nine miles distant from the original discoveries and, later still, on 4 November, a right forearm and hand wrapped in newspaper were discovered.

Among the remains were portions of various newspapers including part of the *Sunday Graphic*, dated 15 September 1935. This was to prove particularly significant as it was a special 'slip' edition of the paper published only in the Lancaster district. Consequently, the attention of the police was immediately directed towards Lancaster and, at the same time, it became known that a Scottish newspaper had reported as missing a Lancaster woman who had disappeared three weeks previously. She was Mary Jane Rogerson, employed as nursemaid in the household of Dr Buck Ruxton who had a medical practice at Lancaster. Rogerson's disappearance had been notified to the police and it seemed a sinister coincidence that the doctor's wife was reported as having left him. Officers contacted Mary Rogerson's stepmother who identified the blouse that had been used to wrap some of the human remains. The garment had a patch under one arm which she had sewn in place for her stepdaughter.

Attention turned to Dr Buck Ruxton, an Indian born in Bombay who had Anglicised his name. He had gained his medical qualifications in India and London and had spent time in the Indian Medical Service. He met his future wife in 1927 and they lived together in London. Although her former marriage was dissolved, she and Ruxton never married. The couple moved to Lancaster in 1930, where he established himself in medical practice at 2 Dalton Square.

Dr Ruxton, it appeared, had asked the Lancaster Borough Police several times for their help in finding his wife. He expressed annoyance at veiled suggestions which he believed were being made in the press connecting the discovery of human remains in Dumfriesshire with her disappearance. 'This publicity,' he informed the Chief Constable, 'is ruining my practice.' He seemed distressed at times, tearfully enquiring if it was not possible to publish a denial that there was any connection between the two occurrences in order to 'stop all this trouble'. Ruxton was arrested on 13 October and charged with the murder of Mary Rogerson, an accusation which he vigorously denied. After several remands, he was also charged with murdering his wife, Isabella.

John Glaister had already been called in to examine the remains of what appeared to be two bodies. After Ruxton's arrest, he visited the house at Dalton Square, Lancaster, with his colleague Dr Gilbert Martin and arranged for a number of articles including pieces of the house itself to be taken to the forensic laboratories at Glasgow for detailed examination. Particular attention was paid to the bathroom, wherein it might be supposed that the bodies had been dismembered for subsequent disposal. Glaister was nothing if not thorough; Item 7 was labelled 'bathroom door', Item 9a, 'linoleum, bathroom floor', Item 23a, 'bath and fittings entire', Item 75, 'trap from waste pipe and bath'. The bathroom at 2 Dalton Square was virtually dismantled in its entirety and removed to his laboratory.

While Glaister and his team were looking for evidence of blood traces on the artefacts taken from Ruxton's home, his colleague at Edinburgh University, Professor James Couper Brash, was attempting to reconstruct the bodies, of which the various remains had once been part. Brash was an anatomist and, from the start, Glaister had been convinced that specialist skills would be required to solve this unusual case. Two large, coffin-like boxes had been constructed at Glaister's instructions to convey the remains from the scene of discovery. The boxes were labelled 'Body No. 1' and 'Body No. 2' and their contents allocated on the basis of the best decisions that could be made on the spot. Of the two likely destinations, Edinburgh or Glasgow, the former was geographically closest and it was there that the grim freight was taken in a police van.

Brash found that Head No. 1 had four complete cervical vertebrae attached to it, while Head No. 2 had five vertebrae attached. The upper portion of trunk found among the remains included two cervical vertebrae so that, on the logic that the body normally had seven cervical vertebrae, he assigned the trunk to Head No. 2. The two sections of spinal column fitted well together and their matching characteristics were confirmed by X-ray. The vertebrae attached to Head No. 1 were generally smaller than those on Head No. 2 which tended to support his judgement about where the trunk belonged.

By a painstaking process of fitting bone to bone and piece to piece in all the possible permutations, the two bodies began to take on some semblance of form. Early on, the anatomical experts had concluded that the dismemberment of the bodies had been carried out by someone with medical and anatomical knowledge. The bodies had been cleanly disarticulated at the joints; there was little damage and no evidence that a saw had been used. The sole instrument used in the dismemberment was a knife.

The nature of some of the mutilation confirmed the use of medical knowledge. An illustration of this was the removal of the larynx from the head of Body No. 2. The size of the larynx is a means of determining the sex of an otherwise unidentified corpse as this structure in the neck is usually a third larger in the male. It was apparent that the person who carried out the dismemberment was using medical knowledge to destroy those parts of his victims' bodies which might aid their eventual identification.

The doctors had agreed at an early stage in their examination that both bodies were female. This was an important point of confirmation for the police in pursuing their case against Dr Ruxton. The final reconstruction of the bodies indicated that Body No. 1 was a woman aged between eighteen and twenty-five years, weighing about 105lb with a height of less than five feet. Body No. 2 was a woman aged between thirty-five and forty-five years, weighing between 126lb and 140lb and with a height of a little less than five feet five inches. These characteristics broadly matched those of the two missing women; Mary Rogerson was aged twenty and Isabella Ruxton, thirty-four years.

Vital though this reconstruction work was, it still fell short of providing positive identification. So the work of medical detection proceeded and the murderer's cunning became ever more apparent. For example, there was a piece of skin missing from the right forearm of Body No. 1 in a position where it was known Rogerson had a distinctive birthmark. Similarly, Body No. 2 had tissue missing from the big toe on the left foot where Mrs Ruxton had a bunion. Casts were made of the feet of the two bodies and tried for size in the shoes of the missing women – they fitted in both cases. Vaccination marks and dental histories were also checked, along with any other individual characteristics that would help to build up the bigger picture.

Fingerprint examination was an obvious means of identification but the mutilated condition of the bodies made this nearly impossible. The fingertips had been completely severed from the hands of Body No. 2, although there was a left hand for Body No. 1. By scouring the house at Dalton Square over an eleven-day period, detectives found matching prints. A number of right hand fingerprint impressions were also found but proved valueless for several weeks until the right hand of Body No. 1 was located by the search team still working in and around the original discovery site. Although badly decomposed and having shed the outer layer of skin, it proved possible to visualise fingerprint impressions on the under layer of skin, or dermis, by means of photography. A perfect match was thus obtained with a thumbprint found at Dalton Square. Glasgow detectives had their work corroborated by the FBI in Washington DC and, thus, were able to satisfy themselves and, ultimately, the court, that Body

No. 1 was Mary Rogerson who at one time had lived in the Ruxton household at Lancaster.

There remained the questions posed by the two heads. While photographs existed of both women, no comparison of skull and portrait had been attempted before in a criminal investigation. Undaunted, Glaister had a life-size print made from the negative still in the portrait photographer's possession. In the original photograph, Isabella Ruxton had been pictured wearing a tiara and a diamante-trimmed evening dress. These articles, which were still available, were used to ensure that the life-size print was true both optically and geometrically. Next, life-size negatives of the skull of Head No. 2 were superimposed on the portrait. The outcome was a stunning match between the two, although John Glaister's conclusion was typically restrained; 'The result convinced us,' he wrote, 'that skull No. 2 could have been that of Mrs Ruxton, but not of Mary Rogerson.'

Applying this technique to Mary Rogerson proved more difficult, mainly due to the lack of a good portrait photograph. There were two snapshots of her, one of which pictured her against a backdrop of an iron gate in a low brick wall. Ascertaining that the location was outside a house in Morecambe, Glaister urged the police to find it and arrange for it to be photographed. His wishes were duly carried out, thereby making it possible to enlarge the young woman's head in the snapshot to life size. The results of superimposing the negative of skull No. 1 on the portrait photograph were less impressive than in the case of Mrs Ruxton but nevertheless showed a close comparison. As Glaister put it, 'We could not say that the skulls were positively those of the dead women. But the probability had been established.'

As the various aspects of the investigation proceeded, there was much toing and froing between Glasgow and Edinburgh. John Glaister noted that the Lancaster police officers at Dalton Square had 'blinked' when he told them he wanted to move whole parts of the house to Glasgow. Because of the intense public curiosity in the case, the blinds of the house were kept drawn so that the investigators could at least work in privacy. The disadvantage of this, as daylight faded, was that at times they were practically working in the dark. This resulted in at least one amusing interlude when a detective working in the house for the first time appeared in a state of panic convinced that he had found a body. While groping in the dark for a light switch in the drawing room his hand had touched the cold features of a marble bust which was part of the furnishings of the room.

Once the interiors of parts of the rooms had been re-assembled in his forensic laboratory at Glasgow University, Glaister had all the time and light he needed to carry out his detailed examinations. His insistence on removing a large section of staircase from the house led to another amusing situation. In order to reach the top of the house, it was necessary to climb a long ladder, stretching almost vertically through three floors. Having ascended to the top with a colleague to work in one of the uppermost rooms, he found himself stranded because it proved impossible to come down without help to guide his feet onto the rungs. As the policemen who were stationed below had gone off to lunch, he had to wait for an hour and a half until they returned.

Having ready access to parts of the rooms reconstructed in his laboratory paid dividends in terms of the detailed examinations he was able to carry out. He tested numerous stains for human blood and found positive results on the stairs and in the bathroom. His report was meticulous. For example, Item No. 9a – 'linoleum, bathroom floor' – consisted of two portions; of his examination of the larger piece, he recorded, 'A. There are two areas of brownish staining situated 9' and 15' respectively from the extreme left end facing bathroom cupboard.' These and general scrapings were removed, labelled 'A', and were submitted to microscopic, chemical and spectroscopic tests for blood pigment with positive results for mammalian blood. They were further submitted to the serological test with positive result giving indication that the blood was human.'

The report signed by John Glaister and Doctors Millar and Martin confirmed that human bloodstains were present throughout the house. They were on and around the bath and hand-wash basin, on and under the bathroom linoleum, on the stairs and banisters, on the stair carpet, on a leather coat belonging to Dr Ruxton, on his wife's corsets and even on the chamber pot in Mary Rogerson's bedroom. Glaister acknowledged that dismembering a human body was a formidable task and he thought that, allowing for a murderer equipped with skill and the proper instruments, eight hours would have been needed to complete the job.

While the doctors had been engrossed in their examinations and tests, the police had been pursuing their side of the investigation which included an analysis of Dr Ruxton's movements and behaviour. It appeared from entries in his diaries that he and Isabella frequently engaged in bitter arguments. There was ample evidence to indicate his jealous and sometimes violent character. He uttered threats and abuse to his wife in the presence of witnesses and had menaced her at various times with both knife and gun. On two occasions, the police were called to the house on account of his explosive behaviour. Isabella had threatened to leave him and he let it be known that she had tried to commit suicide.

Friends and relatives alike believed that Ruxton's jealous attitude bordered on the unbalanced. In early September, a week before she disappeared, Isabella, travelling alone, visited some friends in Edinburgh. They stayed overnight at a hotel and, Ruxton, riven with jealousy, convinced himself that his wife had embarked on an assignation with one of their hosts. Consequently, he followed them in a car in order to satisfy himself on this point. The event passed and, on 14 September, Isabella drove to Blackpool to see the illuminations with her two sisters. She left to return home to Lancaster at about 11.30 p.m. This was the last time that she was seen alive.

Ruxton employed two women to carry out the menial tasks in his house. They normally worked every day of the week but on Friday 13 September the doctor told Mrs Elizabeth Curwen there was no need for her to come back to work until the following Monday. Mrs Agnes Oxley who usually worked on Sundays was informed by a message delivered by her employer to her husband, 'not to trouble to come down this morning'. At about 9 a.m. Sunday morning, the papers were delivered to 2 Dalton Square. The ring on the front door bell summoned not a servant, as expected, but Dr Ruxton himself who appeared to be in an agitated state. Later in the morning, the milkman called and was dealt with by Ruxton and, at 11 a.m. he turned away a woman who had brought her son along by appointment for a minor operation. He explained that his wife was away and that he was busy taking up the carpets in readiness for the decorators. He invited his visitor to see how dirty his hands were. Shortly after 4.30 p.m., he went to the home of one of his patients, Mrs Mary Hampshire, and asked if she would help him prepare the house for the decorators, because he had cut his hand while opening a tin of fruit.

Mary Hampshire returned to the house with Ruxton, where she observed a strange state of affairs. The doors of the bedrooms were locked and the carpets on the stairs had been taken up and deposited in the yard at the rear of the house. One of the carpets was badly stained with blood and there was also a bloodstained shirt and towels. Ruxton explained that he had tried to burn these articles with the aid of petrol. Earlier in the day, he had called in at the local garage and bought four gallons of petrol in two containers. Mrs Hampshire swept the stairs, cleaned the bath and did some washing before returning home. By way of reward Ruxton gave her the stair carpet and a blue suit which he said had become bloodstained when he cut his hand. The next day he called on Mrs Hampshire and asked her to return the suit so that he could have it cleaned. She declined, saying that as he had been generous enough to give her the suit, the least she could do was to clean it herself. After he left empty-handed, Mary Hampshire examined the garment carefully, finding the waistcoat so heavily bloodstained that she burned it. Close examination of the stair carpet also showed it to be damp with blood. She took it out into the yard and sloshed several buckets of water over the stain in her efforts to remove it.

When Ruxton returned to Dalton Square, he found Mrs Oxley waiting. They went into the house together; she made him some coffee and helped him bandage his injured hand. He told her that his wife's visit to Edinburgh was contrived and that she had been aided and abetted in her departure by Mary Rogerson who had asked for her wages in advance. Mrs Oxley noted that the stair carpet had been taken up and that the doors of several of the rooms were locked and the keys were not available. Mrs Hampshire called as arranged at around midday. He confided in her that he was the most unhappy man in the world and that his wife had gone away with another man, leaving him with three children to look after. Bitterly distressed he told her that he could forgive extravagance but not infidelity.

On 17 September when Mabel Smith, the charwoman, arrived at the house, she was instructed by Ruxton to start stripping the wallpaper from the staircase wall in preparation for the decorators. The doors which had previously been kept locked were now open, but the daily help was aware of an unpleasant smell in the house. Both Mrs Smith and Mrs Curwen were told to maintain fires which had been started in the yard. Papers and clothing were burned and Mrs Smith saw bloodstained cotton wool in one of the fires. Several persons passing the house late at night saw the fires still burning and one witness observed Ruxton supervising the conflagration. A day or two later, Mrs Curwen was asked by her employer to buy a spray and a bottle of eau-de-cologne, as he had noticed a stuffy smell in the house. When Mabel Smith began the task of emptying the soiled linen basket, she found a white nightdress with a large bloodstain on it. She took the garment and washed it to remove the stain.

Despite all these strange occurrences at 2 Dalton Square, Ruxton kept up a series of excuses and his servants unquestionably did his bidding; in the process, a great deal of valuable evidence was destroyed. But Ruxton maintained his pretences and, on 24 September, was busily complaining of what today would be termed police harassment. His chief complaint concerned questions asked of his servants about the death of one of his patients. All of this, of course, occurred before the discovery of the remains in Dumfriesshire. When he read a report in the *Daily Express* explaining that part of the remains were those of a male, he turned to Mrs Oxley and said, 'So you see . . . it is a man and a woman; it is not our two.'

Ruxton's edgy behaviour grew worse. On 10 October, he asked Mrs Hampshire about the suit he had given her. She explained that she had it upstairs; 'Do something about it', he said. 'Get it out of the way. Burn it.' He was also worried about the carpets. Later on the same day, he called at the police station and complained that rumours were damaging his practice; 'Can nothing be done to stop this talk?' he asked. He gave the officers a description of his missing wife and also provided a photograph. The next day, he compiled a document called 'My Movements' which listed his comings and goings from 14 to 30 September. He made further complaints to the police about the damaging effects of the current rumours. Referring to a report in the *Daily Express*, which mentioned that one of the bodies had a full set of teeth in the lower jaw, he said, 'I know of my own knowledge that Mary Rogerson has at least four teeth missing in this jaw.' Captain Vann, the Chief Constable, might have been forgiven for thinking that the little doctor 'protested too much'. At any rate, on 12 October, he had Ruxton arrested and placed behind bars, despite his vigorous protests of innocence.

As John Glaister put it, 'Probabilities, possibilities and facts all woven together formed the circumstantial evidence which was the basis of the Crown case when Ruxton's trial began.' He appeared before Mr Justice Singleton at Manchester's High Court of Justice on 2 March 1936. Some figures of future eminence appeared as counsel, including David Maxwell Fyfe and Hartley Shawcross for the prosecution and Norman Birkett for the defence. A worry that Glaister had was that his estimate of between ten and fourteen days as the time which had elapsed since the deaths of Mary Rogerson and Isabella Ruxton and the discovery of their bodies might be seriously challenged in court. He was mindful that, in Norman Birkett, Ruxton had the services of probably the greatest defence lawyer in the country at that time.

Among the many samples and specimens that he had collected at the scene of discovery, Glaister remembered he had obtained some maggots which lay, preserved for posterity, in specimen tubes in his laboratory. It occurred to him that these unpleasant bluebottle larvae might provide a useful indication of dates. In accordance with his usual custom, he sought expert advice by consulting an entomologist at Glasgow University. Dr Alexander Mearns, without any preamble, told him that the stage of development of the larvae showed they were between twelve and fourteen days old.

Elated with what he regarded as unchallengeable evidence, Glaister took his microscope, together with his slides and specimens to Manchester. He presented his new evidence to the Assistant Director of Public Prosecutions and Crown counsel and was amazed, and probably somewhat annoyed, that they rejected his idea of introducing it in court. What concerned the prosecution team was not the validity of Glaister's arguments but of its impact on the jury. It was put to him that jurors who had listened to the most horrific evidence concerning the dismemberment of human bodies might weaken at the prospect of hearing about maggots. The worry was that if a juror went sick and was unable to fulfil his duties, the law as it then stood would require a new trial with a fresh jury. Glaister had to accept the combined wisdom of the prosecution lawyers, albeit reluctantly, but he reserved the right to volunteer the evidence if he found it necessary to protect his reputation.

He was called to give evidence on the seventh day of the trial, as he later described it, 'looking out on benches crammed with a generous representation of members of the Bar, and to the curve of the gallery packed with an array of British and international pressmen'. His evidence was given over two days and his cross-examination by Norman Birkett began late on the first day. 'This was our first encounter,' he wrote, 'and coming under his verbal scrutiny was an experience I'll always remember.' Counsel taxed him on the question of the degree of skill used to dismember the bodies. 'In several cases,' he said, 'there are superficial cuts upon the surfaces of the bones. Is that not also an indication of inexpert and unskilful work?'

'Maybe,' replied Glaister. 'I have often done it myself, and if I were working with haste I would not guarantee that I would not do it. It is just a very tiny injury: the superficial surface of the covering cartilage.'

'Do these matters not indicate that the person who did this was not possessed of any degree of real skill in the matter at all?' asked Birkett.

'I do not honestly think I could subscribe to that view,' replied Glaister.

Counsel also queried the bunion which Mrs Ruxton was known to have on her left foot and its alleged removal as a possible source of identification. 'Is the condition which you found . . . not one which is perfectly common for millions of people, on their feet?'

'It is by no means an uncommon condition,' answered the witness.

'Then all you are able to say,' continued Birkett, 'is that there is no evidence now of what is called bursitis, and that, in your view, there is a malformation which might be the site of a bunion in life?'

'Very possibly: highly possible, the seat of a bunion.'

'You will agree that with millions of people the same thing is to be found?'

'I would not be quite so extravagant as millions,' answered Glaister. 'I would say in a number, of course.'

The expert witness was questioned extensively regarding the bloodstains and their interpretation. It began with the build-up of credentials to which all experts are entitled but which sometimes presages a fall. This was not to be so in Glaister's case but he knew he had to keep his wits about him. 'You have been a very diligent worker in that field, and done a great deal of work upon the tests for blood, and also made your contribution to medical science upon the matter for students and colleagues to work upon?'

'Yes.'

Birkett asked him about the precipitin test and the fact that in the presence of soap it ceased to be reliable. 'Put in words which may be familiar to you,' he said, 'the haze which soap brings is one of the facts which makes it difficult to be sure of the results?'

'Yes', answered Glaister, 'I think that is my own wording.'

Counsel went on to mention the considerable amount of cleaning which had been carried out in Ruxton's house using soap and, in the case of some of the carpets, considerable amounts of water. His point was that the water would have diluted the blood to a degree sufficient to invalidate the testing procedure and that soap used to clean the woodwork of the staircase would have had a similar effect. Glaister defended the reliability of his tests in the circumstances in which he had used them. Pressed by Birkett about the human protein discovered on the eyelets of the stair rod holders and whether it was distinguishable from the soap used to clean them, the witness drew on the immense detail of the investigations he had carried out. He agreed that, had the debris been taken from the surface of the eyelets, it might be similar to soap but, he added, 'the debris was taken from the interior of the stair rod holders, and, I, personally, unscrewed these eyelets before I took scrapings.'

Questioning continued in this fashion, teasing and testing Glaister through a myriad of details of which he showed himself to be the complete master. Turning to the condition of Dr Ruxton's suit, Birkett sought to explain the bloodstains on it by suggesting they resulted from blood splashing during minor operations such as teeth extraction. It was known that Ruxton had on occasions administered anaesthesia in dental surgery. 'In such an operation,' asked Birkett, 'blood, quite naturally, might come upon the suit if it was unprotected by a white overall?' The witness made it clear that there was no arterial spurting of blood in such an operation but he agreed there might be spitting. Counsel suggested that a patient recovering from an anaesthetic very often spits out blood and Glaister agreed. 'And if the anaesthetist was near, he is liable to get some blood upon his coat?'

'Yes,' was the reply from the witness.

Birkett started to move onto weak ground when he extended his arguments. Referring to operations such as circumcision, he said that unless the doctor wore protective clothing he was liable to get spots of blood on the front of his jacket. He went on to say that it would not be possible to say whether all the stains on the jacket in question 'came at one and the same time'. Glaister agreed with this proposition but barely concealed his disgust at the thought; 'I could not conceive of a practitioner,' he said, 'taking part in operative cases with a suit in the condition in which I saw it,' adding, 'it would be a potential source of infection in itself.'

John Glaister's anxiety that he would be pursued on the question of time of death did not materialise. Consequently, the lid was kept firmly closed on his jar of bluebottle maggots. In truth, the case against Ruxton was overwhelming and the scientific evidence was meticulous to the point of perfection. After he had completed his evidence, and with the case at an end, Glaister was invited to dinner by Birkett and they talked in his rooms afterwards, well into the small hours. This was a measure of the distinction which the great defender placed on the professional reputation of the forensic pathologist. In an interview on television years later after he had retired, Birkett was asked whether he had ever defended a person charged with murder whom he knew was guilty. He referred to the Ruxton case in his reply and acknowledged the hopelessness of the defendant's case; 'Nobody could read, as I read,' he said, 'all the facts the prosecution were going to prove without feeling that, well this is a very difficult case.'

All the facts had been assembled through the cooperation of police forces on both sides of the border and by the skill of numerous medical and scientific experts. The case achieved one of John Glaister's ambitions which was to conduct the best possible forensic effort through teamwork. The result of eleven day's presentation of evidence in court was to convince the jury of Dr Buck Ruxton's guilt. He was convicted and sentenced to death, the jury taking sixty-four minutes to reach its verdict.

Surprisingly, in view of the horrific nature of Ruxton's crimes, there were strong petitions in favour of granting a reprieve. Six thousand of Lancaster's citizens signed petitions asking the Home Secretary to intervene. He declined and Ruxton was hanged on 12 May 1936 at Strangeways Prison. In a unique aftermath, on the Sunday following his execution, Ruxton's signed confession was published in the *News of the World*. This was dated 14 October 1935, forty-eight hours after he had been arrested. He sealed the confession in an envelope and entrusted it to one of the newspaper's reporters with instructions that it must not be opened except on his death. He admitted killing his wife in a fit of jealous anger and then killed Mary Rogerson who had witnessed his crime.

The significant part which John Glaister had played in the Ruxton case won him many plaudits and he found himself a sought-after medico-legal property. Like his Edinburgh colleague, Sir Sydney Smith, he was offered the directorship of Lord Trenchard's Metropolitan Police Forensic Laboratory and, like Smith, he turned it down. He disliked the thought of working in London and the prospects for research were not as reassuring as he would have liked. An important follow-up to the Ruxton trial was the publication, with Professor Brash, in 1937, of a book on the *Medico-Legal Aspects of the Ruxton Case*. This was a complete record of the medical and scientific aspects of the investigation which won the Swiney Prize awarded by the Royal Society of Arts. Their use of photo-imposition techniques was an example of pioneering work which found its way into all the forensic medicine textbooks and became a standard procedure in establishing the identity of human remains. In 1942, Keith Simpson made use of the method in his celebrated piece of medical detection in the Dobkin case.

One of his father's achievements which 'Young John' continued was the publication of *Glaister's Medical Jurisprudence and Toxicology*. This textbook was first published in 1902 and appeared in five editions up to 1931 edited by Glaister senior. His son took over the work and expanded it to include new branches of investigation. Not surprisingly, in view of Glaister's particular interests and achievements, the text was particularly authoritative on identification and the examination of bloodstains. Later editions paid special attention to poisons and poisoning. During his lifetime, he saw the textbook through a further eight editions and it was to be frequently cited as a source of authority in the courts. This was entirely proper, for he had few, if any, contemporaries as well qualified in medicine, science and the law – the foundation stones of modern medical jurisprudence.

Like his confrére, Sydney Smith, at Edinburgh, Glaister spent the years of the Second World War at the home front. Apart from the violence which human beings continued to mete out to one another on the domestic front, there were the ravages of enemy action to be overcome. Bomb damage at the University of

Glasgow meant that Glaister was obliged to work from home until it too was damaged during a night-time air raid. He and his wife stayed with friends and he combined his forensic work with fire-watching duties.

The influx of military personnel from a variety of Allied countries and numerous cultural backgrounds, most of them equipped with firearms, meant that it was, as Glaister put it later, 'a time of shooting'. Deaths of soldiers from gunshot wounds had to be investigated to determine whether they resulted from accident, murder or suicide. Many incidents stemmed from drunkenness and the casual handling of firearms. When the USA began sending troops to Britain in preparation for the invasion of Europe, Glaister was asked to extend his practice by taking on forensic cases for the US military. The cultural and social impact created by the appearance of young Americans in British communities has been well documented. What it meant for the forensic expert was to pick up the pieces when the two cultures collided and violence erupted.

Brawls sometimes ended fatally when men with time on their hands before the D-Day invasion had differences of opinion, usually over a girlfriend. Once the circumstances were established, justice was swift and Glaister recalled giving evidence at the court-martial of an American serviceman charged with killing a Polish seaman. There was a scuffle in a Glasgow street when a couple of sailors tried to entice two girls away from their American consorts. In the altercation which followed, one of the GIs was stabbed, causing a slight abdominal wound. The greater injury was to his pride for he acquired a knife and went on a hunt for his assailant. He confronted the Polish seaman in Argyle Street and fatally stabbed him in front of several witnesses.

John Glaister gave evidence at the soldier's court-martial and there was no doubt that he had committed a premeditated killing although, admittedly, he had been provoked. The court, held at the US Army's temporary HQ in a large house in Glasgow's West End, found the man guilty of unlawful killing and he was sentenced to death, a verdict later commuted to life imprisonment. He played no further part in the war effort and was sent back to America to fulfil his prison sentence. A war-time shortage of alcohol in its more acceptable forms proved a challenge to Glaswegians and a steady stream of deaths resulted from improvisation. Compass fluid and aircraft fabric dope were among the substitutes, along with methyl alcohol which was used as an industrial solvent. These concoctions caused respiratory and cardiac failure and added to the pathologists' workload.

As the war in Europe drew to a close, John Glaister had the dubious privilege of being in court for the trial of the only person in Scottish criminal history to be tried twice for murder. Patrick Carraher was a mean man for whom violence was second nature. In August 1938, he had been involved in an argument with three young men and a girl in the Gorbals area of Glasgow. With the argument in full swing, a by-passer decided to intervene, with the laudable intention of pacifying the participants. Carraher drew a knife and slashed the would-be peacemaker across the neck, severing the jugular vein and causing him to bleed to death.

Glaister's post-mortem revealed a deep slash wound which also penetrated the tissues to a depth of two inches. It was the hallmark of a man whose subsequent history showed a great affinity with the knife. On this occasion, owing to a skilful defence, the charge against Carraher was reduced to one of culpable homicide, the Scottish equivalent of manslaughter, and he was given a prison sentence of three years. When he was released in 1941, he was judged unfit to serve his country on account of physical weakness, but he was soon in action with his knife. By 1943, he was serving a further prison sentence for wounding a man with a razor.

In November 1945, Carraher was told of a brawl taking place at a public house in Townhead. By the time he reached the scene, the fight was over and the protagonists had dispersed, although John Gordon, a spectator at the earlier action, lingered nearby. That was his undoing for he was set upon by Carraher who stabbed him in the neck. Gordon, a Seaforth Highlander who had survived the German prisoner-of-war camps, died within minutes of being carried into the Royal Infirmary. Once again, Carraher was tried for murder but, on this occasion, John Glaister was a spectator rather than a participant in court.

As at the first trial, Carraher's counsel sought to prove reduced culpability, pleading diminished responsibility, a defence that in 1946 was only available in Scotland. The grounds were that he was a psychopathic personality whose emotional instability had been aggravated by alcohol and persecution mania. The plea won no converts among the jury who brought in a guilty verdict. In a peculiarly Scottish case, the judge, Lord Russell, pronounced sentence of death on the 'panel', as the accused was called, using an archaic form of words which Glaister noted in his autobiography:

> I decern and adjudge you, Patrick Carraher, panel, to be carried from the Bar to the prison of Barlinnie, Glasgow, wherein to be detained till the twenty-third day of March current, and upon that day, between the hours of eight and ten o'clock forenoon within the walls of the said prison, by the hands of the common executioner, to be hanged by the neck upon a gibbet until you be dead, and your body thereafter to be buried within the walls of the said prison, and ordain your whole movable goods and gear to be escheat and inbrought to His Majesty's use; which is pronounced for Doom.

John Glaister had devoted a great deal of his professional career to the examination of the minutiae of forensic evidence. A murder committed on a Perthshire Farm in 1947 provided clues which were particularly appropriate to his talents

— a few hairs adhering to a discarded safety razor. Catherine McIntyre, the wife of a sheep manager, was found dead in a bedroom of the family home by her son when he returned from work. The room was locked and Archie McIntyre broke down the door with an axe when he realised that something was wrong. His mother had been bound and gagged and suffered severe injuries to her head. A search of the house revealed that money had been stolen and a man's suit was missing from the wardrobe.

Asked by the police to recall any unusual occurrences, Archie McIntyre mentioned that when he left the house in the morning he had noticed a movement in the deep bracken close to the house. He did not hold this to be particularly significant at the time, assuming that the movement was probably caused by an animal. When he pointed out the spot to the police, investigators found a flattened area among the four foot-high bracken which could easily have provided cover for a man. A thorough search of the vicinity quickly turned up a safety razor blade and a piece of bloodstained handkerchief. Later on, a sawn-off, double-barrelled shotgun with bloodstains on its butt was also found in the undergrowth. Close to the gun were two cartridges, a pair of bloodstained overalls and a railway ticket.

This latter discovery provided the first tangible lead. Issued on 25 September 1947, the day before the murder, for a journey from Perth to Aberfeldy, the ticket was of a type issued only to soldiers in uniform. On the shores of Loch Tay and within sight of the farm at which the murder had been committed, was a resettlement centre for Polish troops who had decided to make their future in Britain after the war. At the time, Taymouth Castle was home to 800 Poles and it was there that police began their enquiries.

The breakthrough came when a gardener at Old Meldrum in Aberdeenshire heard a radio report about the killing near Loch Tay in which a description was given of the shotgun found near the scene. He recognised the weapon described as similar to a shotgun he had loaned to a local farm worker. It transpired that the farm worker had reported the gun missing and local enquiries showed that a temporary worker had left at about the same time, stating that he intended looking for a new job in Perthshire. This man was Polish, named as Stanislaw Myszka, who later returned to Old Meldrum wearing a new suit and with money to spend. The farm worker and his wife who had befriended the Pole identified the bloodstained handkerchief found near the McIntyre farm as one they had given to him.

Myszka was traced to a disused RAF camp thee miles west of Peterhead where he had been living rough in one of the huts. He made a run for it when he saw two police officers approaching his lair, but they proved fleet of foot and, after a chase across the fields, they captured him. Among his possessions at the RAF camp were a jacket and waistcoat stolen from the McIntyre home and, when he was searched at the police station, Catherine McIntyre's wedding ring was found in one of his shoes.

After he and a colleague from Glasgow University had carried out a post-mortem examination of Mrs McIntyre's body, Glaister turned his attention to the items found near the scene of the crime. The police produced a safety razor blade with what they thought might be beard hairs stuck to it; they supposed it had been used by someone needing a dry shave. '. . . anything to do with hairs or fibres has always particularly interested me,' wrote Glaister later. 'I'd like to see this blade,' he told the police. The blade was produced and his keen eye took in the few short stubble hairs attached to it. He carefully removed these and placed them in a specimen tube, returning the razor blade to the police for fingerprint examination. Knowing that Myszka was in prison, he asked if it would be possible to obtain some of the prisoner's beard hairs when he shaved in the morning.

In due course, a Perthshire Constabulary vehicle arrived at Glaister's laboratory and a small container was delivered to the professor. In it were a few tiny fragments of hair which soon found their way onto glass microscope slides and thence were subjected to close scrutiny by the world's foremost expert on hair evidence. After comparing the known sample of Myszka's hair with the hairs found on the razor blade, he was satisfied that they matched sufficiently to have come from the same source. He then prepared his findings in readiness to attend as an expert witness for the Crown at Myszka's trial. Glaister knew that he would be severely tested by the defence because, for all its undoubted forensic value, hair evidence lacked the certainty associated with fingerprints.

As he expected, F.C. Wall KC, defence counsel for Myszka, sought to undermine the worth of Glaister's evidence. He suggested that while the hair specimens were similar, they were, 'not too similar to exclude the possibility of it being somebody else's hair altogether?' John Glaister's answer to the question and to the quite proper further probing by the judge, Lord Sorn, was a model of the weight that an expert should put on his professional judgements. He answered, 'We can never say that hair came from the individual unless we take it from the individual,' and acknowledged that, 'As far as we can go is that the characters are so common as to be consistent with a common source.'

The judge made the obvious comparison with fingerprints, pointing out that when similar characteristics are obtained, it is convincing because we know that no two fingerprints are the same. 'Without enlarging greatly,' he asked, 'is there anything of the same nature with regard to hairs?' Glaister replied that comparing fingerprints involved more direct diagrammatic comparison than was possible for hair. Examination of hair was a more complex procedure involving cellular characteristics, both the general and detailed structure and the coloration. 'If we were to take at random a bunch of hair from any one head in this court,' he explained, 'and put them under a microscope we would notice variations in the head hair of the same subject.' He went on to say that by careful examination, it would be possible to find dominant features common throughout such samples, 'it is on that dominating character we do our matching,' he said.

Lord Sorn asked the witness if '. . . you would not go so far as to say that you might not find two identical hairs microscopically from different heads?' Glaister replied, 'I can only say that by matching one sample with another that way, finding the detailed and gross microscopical characters to be identical, it permits us to say they are consistent with a common source. Beyond that I cannot go.' His balanced appraisal of this aspect of the evidence allowed the jury of eleven men and four women to decide what confidence they could place on it.

Despite Mr Wall's special defence that Myszka was not guilty because he was insane and not responsible for his actions at the time of the crime, the jury brought in a guilty verdict. It took them only twenty minutes to reach a verdict and, as Robert Jackson put it in his book *The Crime Doctors*, the additional weight provided by the forensic medical evidence helped the jury to find Myszka guilty. The deserter from the Polish Army in exile was sentenced to death and Albert Pierrepoint carried out his hangman's duty in February 1948.

The satisfaction in this case for John Glaister was not so much in bringing a murderer to justice but in demonstrating the important role of trace evidence in the investigation of crime. He had spent the best part of his career developing methods which would enable forensic scientists to confirm links between criminals and victims. He called these links the theory of interchange and wrote, 'I can't say how the term first came to be used,' but acknowledged the theory, 'has always been one in which I have taken a particular interest.'

The principle of interchange is a simple one; it is that no one involved in a crime departs from the scene without leaving some trace of his presence behind or carrying away some trace which links him irrevocably to the scene. It is the scientific principle underlying Sherlock Holmes's remarkable powers of observation when he was consulted by John Openshaw in 1887 in the case of *The Five Orange Pips*.

'You have come up from the south-west, I see,' observed Holmes.

'Yes, from Horsham,' answered his visitor.

'That clay and chalk mixture which I see upon your toecaps is quite distinctive,' explained the great detective.

The pioneering French criminologist, Edmond Locard, was one of the first investigators to employ scientific methods in this new field. He stated the principle that 'every contact leaves a trace' and demonstrated it in a criminal case in 1912. The trace evidence in question was debris taken from beneath the fingernails of a murder suspect. When Locard examined this under the microscope he found epithelial cells coated with a pink dust which proved to be face powder identical to the cosmetics used by the murder victim. This material had been forced under the murderer's fingernails when he strangled the girl.

'The scientist's task,' said John Glaister, 'is to examine these links which, in crime, can establish a suspect's presence at the scene and occasionally even indicate his actions in relation to the incident'. He illustrated the principle from a case in his own files involving two Glasgow robbers and a bungled attempt to blow a safe. They broke into a carpet warehouse and prepared the safe in the manager's office with explosives and detonator, trailing their wire to a battery at a safe distance. In order to muffle the explosion, they placed some rugs over the safe and, retreating to their refuge, blew the charge. The result was an explosion which, in consequence of being poorly calculated, had not only destroyed the lock but also damaged the safe door so that it could not be opened. In addition, the explosion had caused the rugs to disintegrate, plastering the room with a shower of coloured fibres.

The would-be safe breakers escaped empty-handed but not unmarked. When John Glaister was called in, his eyes no doubt lit up when a detective asked him, 'We wondered whether these fibres might help.' By this time, the police had two suspects in custody and Glaister immediately asked to see their clothes. One set of clothing was clean, indicating that its owner had changed after the attempted robbery, but the other set was a kaleidoscope of trace evidence. There were fibres from the selection of coloured rugs blown to smithereens in the warehouse and traces of powder similar to the explosive used in the incident. As a clinching piece of linking evidence, it was found that a footprint at the warehouse matched the worn-down shoe of one of the men's footwear. His companion had the forethought to change his clothes but not his shoes. Adhering to the heel of the right shoe was a piece of chewing gum in which was embedded a random sample of the myriad of fibres scattered about the warehouse by the explosion. Thus there was ample proof to link both men to the scene of the crime and ample evidence in the hands of John Glaister to convince the court of their guilt. As he wrote later, 'I doubt if it would have consoled them to know that ... they inadvertently furnished university classes with an excellent demonstration of interchange.'

Another kind of interchange occurs as the result of violent contact, for example, during a struggle between victim and assailant or in a hit-and-run incident. In the early hours of 28 July 1950, a Glasgow taxi driver cruising down Prospecthill Road on his way to Kilmarnock, saw the mangled body of a woman lying in the road. His immediate reaction was that she had been run down by a fast-moving vehicle. He called the police and PC William Kevan arrived at the scene.

Kevan was a veteran police officer with over twenty years' service which included experience of investigating many traffic accidents. As he paced the area and looked for the signs normally associated with a hit-and-run incident, he realised that the evidence did not add up. To begin with, he thought the injuries to the woman were far more severe than those normally associated with such incidents. What he found more vexing was the complete absence of any debris at the scene. There was usually broken glass and dirt shaken off the underside of the vehicle when contact was made with a pedestrian. Added to this were curious tyre marks in the road. There were two sets of brake marks and the body lay across them. One set of marks had been made by a vehicle travelling in a westerly direction while the other set, slightly curving, had been made by a vehicle moving in the opposite direction. His suspicions well and truly aroused, PC Kevan called in his CID colleagues.

The post-mortem examination of the victim bore out the constable's initial impression that the incident was not what it seemed. Dr James Irvine and Dr Andrew Allison found gross injuries of a type and extent not normally seen in motor accidents. There were thirty external wounds, together with severe internal injuries, yet only superficial abrasions on the legs. When the doctors discovered that a bruise on the woman's head had been made before she died, while other injuries to the face had been caused after death, the whole incident took on a more sinister aspect. The conclusion to be drawn from the forensic evidence was of a woman probably unconscious from a blow to the head when she was run over and killed; then, once dead, the vehicle was reversed and she was run over a second time. All the tyre marks, which PC Kevan had been astute enough to note on his inspection of the road, were made by the same car, so there was no suggestion that two vehicles were involved.

The dead woman was not identified until a friend, worried by her absence, reported the matter to the police. Catherine McCluskey, a forty-year-old unmarried mother, had left her two children with a friend in order that she could have an evening out; it was an evening that ended in disaster. When Rose O'Donnell identified McCluskey's body in the mortuary, she said, 'She told me she was going out with a bobby.' A neighbour confirmed the dead woman's liaison with a police officer whom she claimed was the father of her three-month-old baby and was expected to pay her maintenance. Corroboration of this came from the Glasgow Assistance Board when an official said McCluskey had applied for assistance after the birth of her second child, but refused to name the father, saying only that he was a policeman.

Suspicion was quickly directed at PC James Ronald Robertson by his fellow officers' observation of his movements. Robertson was unusual among the lowly paid ranks of the police at that time in that he could afford to run his own car. During the course of his duty on the night of 28 July, he absconded for a period, telling a fellow officer, 'I'm off to see a blonde.' When Robertson returned to duty well after midnight, it was noticed that he was perspiring a great deal and looked somewhat dishevelled. He explained his appearance saying that he had to stop to carry out repairs on the exhaust system of his car. One of the last duties he performed on his shift was to record the details of the hit-and-run incident in Prospecthill Road, telephoned in by a divisional officer.

Robertson was questioned the following day and found to be in possession of a number of stolen goods. Asked about Catherine McCluskey, he admitted knowing her and said he had picked her up in his car by prior arrangement and she wanted him to drive her a distance of some fourteen miles to Neilston to stay with a friend. He told her he could not abscond from duty for the length of time it would take to drive to Neilston and back. They argued and he told her to get out of the car. She complied and he drove off; then, having second thoughts, he stopped and reversed the car to go back for her. While reversing along the hundred yards or so that he had travelled, he noticed an increase in the exhaust noise of the car. He stopped, and walking round the car, found Catherine McCluskey trapped beneath it with her clothing caught up in the transmission shaft. He realised that he had accidentally run her down. On finding McCluskey under the car and realising that she was dead, he tried to pull her clear, a task which he found nigh on impossible due to the low ground clearance of the vehicle. Climbing into the driver's seat, he engaged first gear and drew forward slightly with the result that the body dropped free onto the road. He said, 'The hopelessness of the situation seemed to be overwhelming. I started the car up and drove away.' This was the account that Robertson gave to fellow officers and, such was its flimsiness, that he was immediately arrested.

Robertson's lies soon became apparent when his car was examined by officers from the traffic department. The bodywork showed no signs whatever of superficial damage that usually resulted from collision with a pedestrian. The evidence was on the underside of the car in the form of blood and hair, but did it substantiate his account of what had occurred?

This was where John Glaister stepped into the scene. He examined all the artefacts of the incident and came up with his own reconstruction. Robertson's uniform was entirely free of blood which seemed strange in view of his account that he had struggled to free the mangled body from beneath his car. By a strange contrast a heavy, rubber truncheon of a non-regulation type which he had in one of his pockets was slightly bloodstained. Glaister next went along to the garage at police headquarters where Robertson's car was housed. 'I spent several days there,' he said, 'crawling around underneath the car.'

Glaister found nothing to support Robertson's story; there was a complete lack of the evidence of interchange which occurs when a person is knocked down by a motor vehicle. The tyre marks in the road at the scene of the incident, combined with the gross injuries to the victim, told their own gruesome tale. It appeared that McCluskey, already dead or unconscious, lay in the road and was run over from different directions. Thirty-three-year-old Robertson, a policeman for five years, was sent for trial on a charge of murder. He appeared at Glasgow High Court before Lord Keith and was defended by John Cameron KC.

Defence counsel tested Glaister on his medical evidence and, in particular, on the injuries to the victim's legs, Cameron suggested that because a great deal of flesh had been torn from the knees, it was difficult to assess how the injuries had been caused. The Professor's reply was to the effect that the injuries were not to the knees as such but to the inner aspects of the knees and he added rather dryly, 'my experience of the female anatomy is that a woman doesn't stand presenting that part to an oncoming car.' Counsel was at pains to establish the possibility that the victim's death resulted from an accident. He asked Glaister, 'If there is no proof that this woman was laid down insensible in the track of the advancing car, can you in any sense eliminate the possibility of an accident?' Choosing his words with meticulous care, the witness replied, 'To this extent, that it is my opinion that the injuries were caused by a forward motion of the car going at some speed. I do not mean at a colossal speed, but I mean at some appreciable speed, and I think that that was done on more than one occasion.'

This damning assessment plainly ruled out death by accident. Robertson might have got away with his callous act if he had not made the mistake of reversing and then driving forward over his victim again to ensure she was dead. But then he did not understand the principle of interchange which as Glaister noted later, had in this case, 'operated both by its absence and its presence'. James Robertson was found guilty by a majority verdict; eight members of the fifteen-strong jury voted for conviction and seven for acquittal. He was hanged at Barlinnie Prison in December 1950.

Like most medical detectives, John Glaister had his share of poison cases and he was fascinated by the features which put poisoning into a class of its own. He acknowledged that, of all forms of murder, poisoning was both the most cruel and the most difficult to solve. Because poisoning is a crime founded on careful, premeditated planning in which the poisoner, acting alone, takes every precaution to avoid suspicion and escape detection, circumstantial evidence plays an important role. The value of circumstantial evidence has often been derided, usually by defence lawyers, but, equally, its virtues have been praised by various judges. Lord Coleridge described circumstantial evidence as being a mere gossamer thread linking a suspect to a crime, yet it might be strong enough to convict. When circumstances connect closely with each other, they can form a strong web, constituting a level of proof which will satisfy a jury. In a case of poisoning, this type of evidence might be the only kind that has a chance of leading to a successful prosecution.

The knowledge and skill of the forensic pathologist, aided by toxicology and scientific method, can add decisively to the circumstantial evidence available in cases of poisoning. The ease with which symptoms of poisoning can assume the cloak of disease and the apparent reluctance of general practitioners to think of poison in domestic deaths, lent weight to the arguments of those who persuaded

John Glaister to write *The Power of Poison* in 1954. He did so, as he noted in his preface, 'as the result of promptings from several quarters'. He used a number of historical cases to illustrate the difficulties of assessing suspicion of poisoning.

One such case was that involving Eugène Marie Chantrelle, a Frenchman who taught in Edinburgh in the 1860s. The amorous teacher seduced a teenage pupil and he married her when she reached the age of sixteen. Within months she had born her first child and her life degenerated into misery as her husband resorted to beating her and issued threats of greater violence. In October 1877, contrary to her wishes, Chantrelle insured his wife for £1,000, the terms of the policy being that the insurance would be met only in the event of accidental death.

On New Year's Day in 1878, Elizabeth Chantrelle was unwell and retired early to bed. The following morning, the maid found Mrs Chantrelle in some distress. She had been vomiting and the room smelled of gas although the gaslight in the room had been extinguished. Chantrelle, who was sleeping in the nursery with the three children, was called to attend to his wife. He remarked that something was wrong with the gas supply and, after opening the window, went off to fetch a doctor. While the master was out of the house, the maid noticed a plate containing pieces of an orange and grapes, together with a tumbler partly filled with lemonade, on Mrs Chantrelle's bedside table. Later that morning Chantrelle told her he had drunk the lemonade and asked her to wash the empty glass.

Chantrelle was absent for about half an hour and, when he returned, he was on his own. A short while later, Dr Carmichael arrived and examined the patient who he believed to be suffering from coal-gas poisoning. He decided a second opinion was needed and sent for Dr Harvey Littlejohn, the city's police surgeon and also a toxicologist. The two medical men believed Mrs Chantrelle was dying and arranged for her to be admitted to hospital where she succumbed soon after arrival.

Littlejohn noticed the smell of gas as soon as he entered the bedroom and asked Chantrelle about it. 'That's the difficulty, I can't make out,' was the reply. When the dead woman was subjected to post-mortem examination, there were none of the usual signs associated with coal-gas poisoning and blood tests proved negative. What was of diverting interest was Littlejohn's conclusion, having seen the woman while still alive, that her symptoms were more consistent with opium poisoning. This view was substantiated by the traces of the narcotic in the vomitus on the bedclothes. But no opium was found in the stomach, although there were the remains of fruit eaten some time before death.

The whole of Edinburgh's medico-legal fraternity became fascinated by the mystery of Elizabeth Chantrelle's death and the French teacher found himself up against a formidable array of forensic expertise when he was tried for murder in the High Court of Justiciary.

Littlejohn reported that the stain on the bedclothes contained about three-quarters of a grain of opium which was nearly a poisonous dose. He had experimented by mixing opium and lemonade and found that the cordial had little effect on the taste of the mixture. He had found opium and other drugs in Chantrelle's house and it was known that the Frenchman had bought extract of opium from a druggist in the city. Dr Douglas Maclagan, Professor of Medical Jurisprudence at Edinburgh University, examined Mrs Chantrelle when she was admitted to hospital and did not think she was suffering from coal-gas poisoning. He believed the signs were more indicative of narcotic poisoning.

The university's Professor of Chemistry, Dr Crum Brown, and Professor of Materia Medica, Thomas Fraser, added their testimony to the investigation of Mrs Chantrelle's death. They endorsed their colleagues' opinions and Crum Brown experimented with various preparations of opium to see if he could duplicate the staining effect found on the bed linen. He concluded that the most likely form of opium used was the solid or semi-solid variety.

All the experts agreed that Mrs Chantrelle had died as the result of narcotic poisoning. It looked therefore as if the leak of coal gas was either coincidental or a deliberately contrived diversion. That it was the latter was proved by employees of the Edinburgh Gas Company who examined the gas supply in the house. The gas bracket on the mantelpiece of the bedroom which appeared to be the only source was functioning perfectly. The gas supply was turned off at the meter when the fitter inspected the house. The meter was working normally and, turning on the supply, the fitter returned to the bedroom where he immediately noticed an escape of gas, but not from the mantelshelf bracket. Closely examining the room, he found a place near the window frame where a gas bracket had been removed. There was a fractured pipe between the woodwork and the wall. Lying on the window ledge was a section of gas pipe which fitted the gap in the supply pipe.

As John Glaister wrote in his account of this unusual case, 'The evidence, considered as a whole, was entirely circumstantial, and the unification of the links, when finally made to form an unbroken chain which established the guilt of the prisoner in the minds of the jury, must surely be considered instructive by those who have an interest in criminology.' Suffice it to say that the jury found Chantrelle guilty by a unanimous decision and he was subsequently hanged for his crime. The case was certainly instructive in bearing out the maxim of forensic medicine that things are not always as they seem. The affair also highlighted the quality of Scotland's forensic system, particularly the willingness, later pursued by Glaister, to draw in experts from other disciplines.

Another Scottish case in *The Power of Poison* and one which drew together Glaister himself and Sydney Smith as expert witnesses for the prosecution was the Oxgang Farm affair. Mrs Margaret McMillan was charged with both attempted murder and murder in a case of arsenic poisoning. The victim was her husband, thirty-nine-year-old Robert Brennan McMillan, who died on 6 January 1940 at his Dunbartonshire farm after a period of gastric illness. McMillan had a history of illness going back to 1937 when his mother noticed his yellow colour which she attributed to jaundice. He also suffered from gastric upsets and neuritis.

Mrs McMillan senior visited her son in the presence of his wife on 3 January 1940 when he complained that his throat was raw down to his stomach. He vomited twice while she was there and she sought reassurance from her daughter-in-law that if he became worse she could call her. On 5 January, she received a telephone message informing her that the doctor on his visit that day had given a satisfactory report on her son. Robert McMillan died the next day. Eleven grains of arsenic were found in his stomach and intestinal tract.

It was known that McMillan had used arsenic around his farm for killing rats. An acquaintance who worked at a glass factory where arsenic was regularly used in large quantities as part of the processing, obtained 2 or 3lb of the poison, which he handed in a paper bag to McMillan. One night, in March 1937, he helped the farmer lay poison traps by spreading the arsenic on slices of bread and placing them strategically around the farm. In December 1939, he supplied Mrs McMillan with about 1lb of arsenic, which he took from the large storage drum at the glassworks. She had complained about rats in her bedroom and he supplied the poison at her request. Following Robert McMillan's death, and the news that his friend had been poisoned, he called at the farm and spoke to the widow. He expressed his anxieties about having to answer questions from the police and she told him there was nothing to worry about. When he enquired specifically about the quantity of arsenic he had given her, she told him that McMillan had flushed it down the drain.

Francis Hughes, the head pigman at Oxgang Farm, made it known that he had been asked to dispose of a bottle of white arsenic powder by throwing it into the River Clyde. He was given this task while Mr McMillan was ill in bed and was told that the bottle contained arsenic. During his employer's illness, Hughes helped him when he wanted a bath because his mobility was affected. He asked McMillan the cause of his illness and was told that he had been mixing arsenical rat poison. Apparently undaunted by the implications, Hughes kept the bottle of arsenic for his own use in killing rats and even supplemented it by asking the McMillans' supplier for more.

Margaret McMillan appeared on trial in June 1940 before the Lord Justice Clerk, Lord Aitchison. John Glaister and Sydney Smith, both veteran investigators of arsenical poisoning cases in Egypt, gave medical evidence. Glaister believed that the symptoms of McMillan's illness in 1937 were consistent with arsenical poisoning and he believed that all of the arsenic ingested at that time would have been excreted from the body well before his death three years later. Consequently, the arsenic found at post-mortem must have been ingested nearer to the time of death and his estimate was within a four-month period.

His basis for this estimate was an examination of the dead man's hair and fingernails which showed arsenic passing out of the body over that period. He believed that the clinical picture over the last two weeks of life was fully consistent with arsenical poisoning and thought that a massive quantity of arsenic had been ingested in one or more doses within twenty-four hours of death. This conclusion was based chiefly on finding 2.33 grains of arsenic in the liver and 11.06 grains in the stomach and intestines. Asked by the Solicitor-General if the arsenic might have entered the body accidentally, Glaister replied, '. . . if one adopted this thesis, the accident must have been oft repeated and repeated over a long interval of time.' On the question of suicide, his opinion was that it would be difficult to understand a person intent on suicide dragging out the process over such a long time.

Glaister was asked if he could give an estimate of the times when, 'arsenic may have got into that man's body,' as the Solicitor-General quaintly phrased it. The expert witness repeated his earlier statement that the terminal illness presented a clinical picture of arsenical poisoning with indications of a rally on 5 January, followed by a rapid deterioration in the early hours of the following morning. His opinion was that, after McMillan took to his bed on 29 December, there were one or more doses of arsenic ingested up to 5 January with a further massive dose or doses within the last twenty-four hours of life. At this point, the Lord Justice Clerk intervened to press John Glaister on the possibilities for explaining McMillan's death due to either accident or suicide. Lord Aitchison asked, 'Supposing the facts in this case show – I ask you to assume – that this man had been getting arsenic into his system to an extent to make him seriously ill, off and on, over a period of months, would that fit in with any case of suicide that you have heard of?'

'No,' came the witness's reply.

'So far as you know,' continued the judge, 'has there been any case in which a man has sought to take his own life, prolonging the agony for a period of months?'

'No,' answered Glaister.

Asked by the judge if, in his experience, the witness had ever encountered a case of accidental poisoning by arsenic which continued over a period of months, John Glaister answered once more with an emphatic 'No.'

Sydney Smith supported the opinion of his forensic colleague and it was left to Lord Aitchison to sum up for the jury which he did at some considerable length. He began by telling them there were occasions when human life was taken in which it was open to a jury to say that something less than murder had been committed. But, he was quick to point out, not in this case. The law would not permit an intermediate verdict of guilty of culpable homicide; the only possible verdicts were 'Guilty' or 'Not Proven'. He acknowledged that poisoning was a secret crime and one that was difficult to detect, although that did not absolve the Crown from the requirement to prove it, relying on circumstantial evidence if necessary.

Having set the working limits for the jury's deliberations, the judge went on to review the evidence. It was undisputed, he said, that Mrs McMillan's husband had died of arsenical poisoning, the poison entering his body during the four to six months prior to his death. The medical evidence had shown with certainty that a massive dose of arsenic had been ingested within twenty-four hours of death. The question was, how did the fatal quantity enter his body; voluntarily, accidentally or by an act of deliberate poisoning on the part of someone else with the intention of killing him. 'If he was murdered, was he murdered by the accused?' asked Lord Aitchison, and continued, 'Now, unless the Crown can prove the third of these propositions, that the late Mr McMillan was murdered, and murdered by the accused, unless the Crown can prove that and prove it satisfactorily, then you are bound to acquit.'

In his review of the medical evidence, the judge said all the experts agreed that McMillan had been ingesting arsenic for at least four months prior to his death. It was clear too that the doses had increased towards the end of his life with two large doses during the final weeks. 'There is no doubt,' said Lord Aitchison, 'that man had got into his system a fatal dose of arsenic.' The question was how did he get it?

Acknowledging his awareness of history, His Lordship made a reference to the trial of Madeleine Smith for murder by arsenical poisoning, 'in this very courtroom.' He quoted part of the judge's charge to the jury on that occasion in 1857, in which he stressed that whatever doubts there may have been about her defence, the evidence against her must be convincing and with no room for conjecture. Echoing the verdict of their predecessors eighty-three years before, the jury gave the benefit of doubt to Margaret McMillan by finding the charges against her 'Not Proven'.

It was said after the Oxgang Farm trial that John Glaister considered omitting the chapter on arsenical poisoning from his book on forensic medicine on the grounds that, 'there will never be another case.' He was nearly right, for there were only two further convictions during his lifetime – Sergeant Marcus Marymont in 1958 and William Waite in 1970.

His purpose in giving accounts of a number of murders by poisoning in *The Power of Poison* was to explore the difficulties of assessing the evidence in such cases. He was aware of the power of circumstantial evidence but emphasised the wide gulf which existed between the apparent evidence of guilt and legal proof. Science could play what he described as a supporting role in the work of criminal investigation. He warned of the need for the scientific expert to keep an open and unbiased mind – a theme to which he returned many times.

In his book, *Final Diagnosis*, Glaister remarked on the differences between English and Scottish practices in the investigation of crime. In England, it was a three-part system, involving the police, a Home Office laboratory scientist and a forensic pathologist. Whereas, in Scotland, the roles of the scientist and pathologist were combined. Glaister was perhaps uniquely qualified for this task with his qualifications as a doctor, scientist and barrister.

Throughout his career, he was an exponent of the need for forensic pathologists to draw on expertise outside their own disciplines. Forensic science had moved quickly since Spilsbury's day so that the role of the self-reliant expert was no longer tenable. Glaister had always shown his willingness to call in other experts and to work closely with them as he had demonstrated in his close cooperation with Professor Brash, the anatomist, in the Ruxton case.

He advocated a unified medico-legal institution for the United Kingdom which would bring together all the essential elements of diverse professional disciplines, with their expertise and experience, under one form of management. He presaged the theme echoed later by Francis Camps and both men left a lasting legacy in the university departments of forensic medicine which they established as prototypes for the future, Glaister at Glasgow and Camps in London.

In the twenty-first century, these concepts of integrated expertise and forensic management would reach fruition in the shape of the multi-disciplined crime laboratory in which crime scene evidence could be comprehensively processed and examined. John Glaister's meticulous archives of mammalian hair samples, recorded in albums of photo-micrographs, would be transformed by computer technology into digitised images available for instant comparison with trace evidence.

It was a progression which epitomised Glaister's *raison d'être* which was that every crime left a trace, however faint, which would lead investigators to the perpetrator. He wrote, '... every year that passes, the skills of forensic medicine are growing, its new techniques are probing forward.' The evolution of forensic science has justified his optimism. He quoted Ralph Waldo Emerson, the American poet and essayist, who wrote, '... there is no den in the wide world to hide a rogue.'

John Glaister retired in 1962 and relinquished his chair as Regius Professor. Thus ended an era in which Glaisters, father and son, had served as successive professors at Glasgow University for sixty-five years. It had been a period of immense advancement on which both Glaisters left their impressive pioneering stamp. In retirement, Glaister continued to lecture, passing on the fruits of his learning to a new generation, and he also worked for the community by being elected a County Councillor.

He died in hospital in 1971 at the age of seventy-nine. Perhaps, inevitably, the obituaries laid emphasis on the father and son succession. *The Glasgow Herald*, in its appreciation published on 5 October 1971, noted that, 'Their continuous period of service must be one of the longest given by one family to a single university.' At the memorial service held in the university chapel, he was remembered as a 'kindly, soft-hearted man' who always had time for conversation.

Chapter Four

THE MENTOR

Francis Camps

PEERING OVER HIS HALF GLASSES, with a pipe in his mouth and a forensic artefact in his hands, Francis Camps epitomised the popular approach to his subject. He enjoyed publicity where other pathologists preferred to shun it. A newspaper headline declaring 'Inquest on a woman who died 5,000 years ago: Dr Camps Investigating', was typical of his involvement. This particular report concerned a skull found in 1962 at a Stone Age Settlement in Middlesex. The newspaper reported that the 'famous pathologist' was subjecting the remains to the full 'forensic treatment'.

Camps also courted controversy during his career by embracing views which antagonised his contemporaries; deliberately, according to some critics. He liked to challenge established views and, to that extent, was something of a maverick. In common with many of the great vocational callings, forensic pathology has its moments of professional jealousy. As its chief practitioners were frequently called upon to perform in public, this was probably inevitable. Spilsbury, the loner, was aloof to criticism, Smith was genuinely a public figure and Glaister was essentially a back-room boy. Camps and Simpson represented the last of their kind in a changing profession where individual flare was giving way to teamwork and technology. Perhaps sensing that the age of the great medical detective was coming to an end, they both wanted to make their mark, first as collaborators and then as rivals.

Francis Edward Camps was born on 28 June 1905 at Teddington, Middlesex, where his father had built up a successful medical practice. Francis was the only one of old Dr Camps's three sons who followed in his father's footsteps by choosing a career in medicine. He also, it seems, followed his father's inclination for confrontation. Dr Camps senior had a reputation for being somewhat cantankerous, although he had a shrewd bedside manner with his wealthy patients. Francis proved to be an individual with restless energy and an enormous capacity for work.

He studied at Marlborough College and the University of Neuchatel in Switzerland before qualifying as a doctor at Guy's Hospital in 1928. After working as a house physician at Guy's, he moved on to the School of Tropical Medicine at the University of Liverpool to take further qualifications. Like many young doctors, Camps could not decide whether to go into general practice or to specialise. He perhaps had a notion that, equipped with a diploma in tropical medicine, he might seek an appointment in the British Colonial Service.

Despite the lure of overseas travel, Camps went into general practice at Chelmsford and spent part of his time at Chelmsford and Essex Hospital. With his indefatigable appetite for work, he coped easily with two jobs and very quickly became the hospital's honorary pathologist. Having drifted into the field of pathology, he decided in 1935 to specialise in this subject. The Essex Police began to seek his advice in crime investigation work and, so, he began to lay the foundations for his later reputation. Camps was rejected for military service because he was insufficiently fit, although he worked as consultant pathologist to the emergency medical services while continuing to be based at Chelmsford.

As Sir Bernard Spilsbury's domination began to wane, the way was clear for a successor. Camps gravitated to London where he encountered Keith Simpson who was based at Guy's and Donald Teare working from St George's with whom he shared the pathology cases. They were often referred to as 'The Three Musketeers', but that was in the early days before a keen sense of rivalry took hold.

In 1945, London Hospital Medical College set up a department of forensic medicine and appointed Francis Camps to run it with the status of lecturer. This gave him a firm base and he quickly set about devoting his energies to building up what came to be acknowledged as one of the foremost centres of forensic medicine. He had the vision to realise that traditional morbid anatomy allied to self-educated detective work was not enough. His ambition was to modernise forensic medicine by bringing together specialists from many different disciplines and at the same time to revitalise academic training methods.

His single-mindedness often left others trailing in his wake and his modest requirements for sleep were almost legendary. He despised tiredness and illness and often worked late into the night either in the laboratory or post-mortem room. Many of those who worked with him admired his energy but also found his personality wearing. Conversation with Camps was usually a monologue, with him doing the talking, and he tended to be demanding and unforgiving. Some of his colleagues, and a number of his peers, found him a difficult man to deal with. And there were those who thought he tried too assiduously to gain public recognition. Whatever the shortcomings of his temperament, there was no doubting his capability as a forensic pathologist. He set a personal example of a high work rate and surrounded himself with talented people. He also had the knack of the gifted organiser who could persuade those in authority to accede to his requests. This earned him a reputation for 'empire building' at London Hospital and he did not endear himself to Keith Simpson by boasting that he had established an unequalled forensic service.

In the immediate post-war years, Camps worked closely with Sir Bentley Purchase, the St Pancras coroner, and the two men became close friends. The North London coroners' circuit provided ample work for Camps and other pathologists. Most of it was routine; the investigation of suspicious remains and death in questionable circumstances. As all pathologists must, Camps had his fair share of rotting human remains to examine and also the victims of fatal violence.

The 1950s saw the beginnings of Camps's rise as a public figure. First, came the case of the torso found in the Essex Marshes, a discovery which prompted large newspaper headlines. On 21 October 1949, Sidney Tiffin was enjoying a wild fowling excursion in Dergie Marshes, Essex. The area of wetland north of the Thames Estuary was a desolate haven for wildlife, relatively free from human intrusion. As he moved about among the reeds, Tiffin spotted a bundle floating in the water. His first thought was that it was a drogue parachute from an RAF training plane, so he ignored it. Later, he had second thoughts and reasoned that it might be worth his while retrieving the chute and returning it to the RAF.

On closer inspection, the bundle turned out to be a felt-covered package secured with rope. His curiosity aroused, Tiffin cut the wrappings and to his horror revealed a headless human torso clothed in shirt and pants. The head and legs were missing and the hands were fastened together with a leather strap. Hastily covering the grisly remains and securing them to a stake driven into the mud to mark their location, Tiffin rushed off to fetch the police. Two police constables guided by Tiffin retrieved the bundle and took it to St John's Hospital mortuary at Chelmsford. Chief Superintendent G.H. Totterdell, Head of Essex CID, immediately sent for Dr Camps. The two men knew each other well and Essex was very much the pathologist's parish, although he was acting in his capacity as Home Office pathologist.

Camps carried out a post-mortem examination from which he concluded that the torso, which was male, had been dismembered using a sharp knife and a saw. Cause of death was due to five stab wounds in the chest. Judging from the external appearance of the remains, he thought the torso might have been in the water for about twenty-one days. The nature of the post-mortem injuries, including multiple rib fractures and damage to the spine, indicated that the torso might have been dropped from a height. In order to determine the identity of the victim, fingerprint impressions were needed. Totterdell described how Camps removed the entire skin of the hands by making an incision around the wrists and peeling it off like a pair of rubber gloves.

Looking at the dark pigmentation of the skin, the detective was fairly certain the remains were those of Stanley Setty, a London businessman who had been reported missing. He was an Iraqi by birth who worked as a car dealer. When he went missing on 4 October, he was carrying £1,000 in £5 notes, the proceeds of car sales. Totterdell told Camps, 'I think we've got Setty's torso here.' His intuition proved correct when Chief Superintendent Fred Cherrill, Scotland Yard's fingerprint expert, reported back to Totterdell, 'It's Setty all right.'

Further searches were made in the Essex Marshes in the hope of finding the head and legs to match up with the torso. A breakthrough in the investigation came soon after news of the discovery of the torso was reported in the newspapers. The activities of a civilian pilot at the United Services Flying Club at Elstree had been observed by airport workers who judged them to be suspicious. Brian Donald Hume had hired an Auster light aircraft the day after Setty went missing and took off for Southend carrying two bulky parcels of airfreight. When he returned, there was some damage to the aircraft which was duly noted.

Hume was sought for questioning and tracked down on 26 October. In answer to police questioning, he said that he had been paid to dispose of parts of a printing press used for counterfeiting petrol coupons. He explained that three men had arrived at his flat and delivered the parcels. Bloodstains were apparent on the carpet in the living room which was taken as evidence of violence and Hume was charged with murder. He appeared on trial at the Old Bailey in January 1950 when Camps gave expert testimony for the prosecution and Dr Donald Teare appeared for the defence. Camps described how Setty had met his death as a result of shock and haemorrhage caused by multiple stab wounds to the chest.

Considerable quantities of blood had been found at Hume's flat and there were varying theories as to its origin. The prosecution believed Setty was murdered there, despite the lack of any fingerprint evidence, and clearly implicating Hume. Against this was the suggestion that Setty had been killed elsewhere and his parcelled-up remains, leaking blood, were delivered to Hume's flat by the three men he had spoken about. The two pathologists did not agree about the bloodstains and there were strong arguments in favour of more than one attacker being involved in the murder.

The jury could not agree a verdict, with the result that Hume was discharged. A new jury was sworn in but the prosecution declined to present any evidence. In consequence, the judge instructed that Hume be found not guilty on the murder charge. He admitted being an accessory to the fact and was sentenced to twelve years' imprisonment. Soon after he was released in 1958, and in the knowledge that he could not be charged again with the same crime, Hume made a confession. His medium was a Sunday newspaper which carried the headline, 'I killed

Setty . . . And Got Away With Murder'. No doubt that is what Francis Camps believed when the trial concluded.

Hume continued to lead an adventurous life, and after he went to live in Switzerland, he shot and killed a taxi driver in the course of a bank raid in Zurich. The Swiss had no difficulty in finding him guilty and he was sentenced to life imprisonment. Sent back to Britain in 1976, he spent the rest of his days at Broadmoor where he died in 1988.

In March 1953, a discovery was made at Notting Hill, London that precipitated one of the most sensational post-war murder investigations. A Jamaican man, newly arrived in Britain, rented a flat at 10 Rillington Place. He was given permission by the landlord to use a ground-floor kitchen because the tenant had absconded. While inspecting the state of the kitchen, the new tenant tapped on one of the walls, which sounded hollow. His curiosity was roused when he realised that he had found a cupboard which had been wall-papered over. When he peeled the paper back and opened the doors, he discovered the bodies of three women holed up in the confined space.

Camps's biographer records that on the evening of 24 March, as he was about to start dinner, the pathologist was called by the police to 10 Rillington Place. The three corpses he saw there were taken to the mortuary at Kensington for closer examination. Camps worked through the night and his burden was added to the next morning after police searches at the house turned up a fourth body concealed beneath the floorboards in one of the bedrooms. The corpses found in the kitchen were all identified as prostitutes; women in their mid-twenties known to the police. The fourth body was that of Ethel Christie, wife of John Reginald Halliday Christie, the missing tenant from 10 Rillington Place. While Camps was absorbed with the grisly task of determining how these women had died, police searching the garden found further human remains. The pathologist would eventually piece together the skeletons of two females who had lain in the ground for nearly ten years. A newspaper found in their grave was dated 19 July 1943.

A manhunt ensued to find John Christie, a fifty-five-year-old office worker, well known in the neighbourhood, who had rented the ground-floor flat at Rillington Place for fourteen years. Meanwhile, Camps proceeded with his examinations and determined that the three bodies walled up in the kitchen cupboard had not been there very long, probably only a matter of months. All three corpses were remarkably well preserved, accounted for by Camps who said the cupboard was dry and well ventilated and the weather had been cold. He determined that the women had been strangled and he found high levels of carbon monoxide in their blood. His conclusion was that they had been gassed, then strangled and subjected to sexual intercourse, either before, during or after death. In the case of Ethel Christie, aged fifty-four, cause of death was strangulation with no evidence of gas poisoning.

A week after the discoveries at 10 Rillington Place, on 31 March, John Christie was arrested on Putney Bridge by a police officer who recognised him from descriptions that had been circulated. While he was being questioned, Camps and his team continued their forensic examination of the remains found in the garden. Working at the London Hospital Medical School under the direction of Professor Richard Harrison, he established the ages of the two women, one being about twenty-one and the other in her thirties. The skull of the second woman was missing from the garden grave, although, in a bizarre resolution of the mystery, it became known that the relic had been unearthed in 1949 by Christie's dog whose master threw it into a bomb-damaged house where it was found by children and eventually brought to the notice of the police who destroyed it. The pathologist paid particular attention to the jawbone belonging to the first set of remains, which contained a tooth crowned in a manner suggesting German or Austrian dental work. The remains were subsequently identified as those of twenty-one-year-old Ruth Fuerst, an Austrian refugee.

Christie made several detailed statements in which he admitted murdering the six women whose bodies had been found, including the strangulation of his wife. He also confessed to the murder in 1949 of Beryl Evans, whose body, together with that of her baby, had been discovered beneath the floor of the wash-house at 10 Rillington Place. Her husband, Timothy Evans, first confessed to the crimes and then blamed Christie who appeared as a witness at his trial for murder. The twenty-six-year-old van driver was found guilty of killing his child and was sentenced to death. He was hanged on 5 March 1950.

Now, in light of what had been revealed at Rillington Place, and Christie's admission that he had killed Beryl Evans, it was decided to exhume the bodies of Beryl and baby Geraldine. This was another grim task allocated to Francis Camps. The exhumation took place on 18 May 1953 at the Roman Catholic cemetery of the Royal Borough of Kensington. Camps conducted the post-mortems aided by Donald Teare who had performed the original examinations in 1949, and Keith Simpson, who was present at the request of Christie's lawyers. As Simpson put it in his autobiography, 'Once, and only once, we three were "on the job" together.' His account of what followed indicated a less than fraternal atmosphere. Simpson was intent on finding possible signs of carbon monoxide in Mrs Evans's body which, if evident, would have been indicative of Christie's method of killing.

The three men gathered around the mortuary table observed pink discolouration of the thighs, a tell-tale sign of carbon monoxide poisoning. Simpson told Camps he wanted tissue samples taken for laboratory analysis and Donald Teare concurred. Camps appeared to be put out by this request and replied, 'I'm in charge here. I'm going to do this my way.' He said he would hand over all the specimens to Dr Lewis Nickolls, Director of the Metropolitan Police Laboratory. The cause of death was pinpointed as asphyxia, thereby confirming Dr Teare's original findings. The laboratory tests proved negative for carbon monoxide and Simpson and Camps agreed that a pathologist of Teare's experience would not have missed evidence of carbon monoxide poisoning if it had been apparent at the original post-mortem.

Among the weird discoveries made at 10 Rillington Place was a tobacco tin containing four tufts of pubic hair. These were presumed to have been taken by Christie from his victims and kept as trophies. Keith Simpson devoted several paragraphs in his memoirs to discussion of the pubic hair which Christie claimed had come from his wife and the three women whose bodies ended up in the cupboard. Microscopic examination did not support this contention, so the origin of the hair remained a mystery. In any event, Camps was not too fussed about this diversion.

The odious former special policeman, John Christie, was tried for the murder of his wife. Outwardly a respectable, though unpopular man, he had served prison sentences for theft and was an habitual liar. He was known as 'Reggie-no-dick' on account of his sexual inadequacy. In evidence, he related how he invited women to his flat, got them drunk and then placed them in his infamous deck-chair where he rendered them unconscious with coal gas. Once they were insensible, he strangled and raped them. He admitted killing Beryl Evans but denied harming her baby. There was little doubt that Timothy Evans was an innocent man caught up in his own false confession. Following Mr Justice Brabin's public enquiry in 1966, the Queen granted Evans a posthumous pardon. By then, Christie had long since met his fate on the scaffold at Pentonville in July 1953.

The ghoulish events which occurred at 10 Rillington Place have been thoroughly chronicled, most notably by Ludovic Kennedy in his book published in 1961. And Richard Attenborough's creepy portrayal of Christie in the 1971 film about the murders was memorable. John Eddowes published an account in 1994 and made the case for two killers at Rillington Place, Evans and Christie. The Attorney-General who prosecuted at Christie's trial, made a point afterwards of commending Francis Camps and his colleagues for their professional skills in dealing with difficult forensic materials. He suggested that the evidence gathered represented a remarkable feat of investigation to which Camps answered, 'I think it is very satisfactory.' A further commendation came from the Director of Public Prosecutions, Sir Theobald Mathew, extending his gratitude to the pathologist and his team for their brilliant work. Camps published his own account of the forensic investigation in his book, *Medical and Scientific Evidence in the Evans and Christie Cases* (1953). He also had the last word on Christie on whose body he carried out the customary post-mortem following execution at Pentonville Prison. He noted, ironically, that 'Reggie-no-dick' has a 'well-developed' penis. Commenting on the conviction of Timothy Evans, he observed that the case was particularly controversial and, 'undoubtedly aided the abolition of the death penalty'.

In November 1953, an event occurred in Germany involving a British service-man that would, in due course, embroil Francis Camps in another sensational case. In the meantime, he continued his far from humdrum professional work with the investigation of the murder of a woman whose burning body attracted the attention of neighbours on 28 July 1954. When the police arrived at the scene in South Hill Park, Hampstead, they found the naked body of Hella Christofi in the garden, charred and reeking with the smell of paraffin.

Camps's examination was straightforward. He found an area of unburned skin encircling the woman's neck with the marks of a knot plainly indicating a liga-ture. She proved to have been strangled with her son's scarf, the remains of which had been thrown into the dustbin. The dead woman had been murdered by her mother-in-law out of obsessive jealousy. Fifty-three-year-old Styllou Christofi, an illiterate woman of peasant origins, had been tried and acquitted in Cyprus, twenty-three years previously on a murder charge. At the Old Bailey in 1954, she declined to plead insanity and evoked little public sympathy. She was convicted of murder and hanged at Holloway Prison.

The following year, after startling developments in the death of a British ser-viceman in Germany, Camps was asked to supervise an exhumation at Cologne. On 30 November 1953, Sergeant Reginald Watters, based at the REME Technical Training College in Duisberg, was found hanging from the banisters in a barrack room stairwell. He had, it seemed, committed suicide. The body, suspended by a rope and with an upturned bucket lying nearby, was found by fellow non-commissioned officer, Sergeant Frederick Emmett-Dunne and another NCO. A post-mortem examination was carried out by a junior pathologist seconded to the British Army on the Rhine. Dr Alan Womack found bruising on the dead man's neck and noted that the thyroid cartilage was broken. On the basis of this report and noting the circumstances in which the body had been found, an army inquest into Sergeant Watters's death returned a verdict of suicide.

The untimely end of a popular NCO was the talk of Duisberg and it was not long before the rumour mills started up. Watters was married to a local German woman and, ostensibly, Emmett-Dunne was his friend. But there was talk of jeal-ousy on Watters's part, who believed his friend was making a play for his wife. For his part, Emmett-Dunne was not popular among his peers who regarded him as arrogant and overbearing. He was also a man of questionable honesty who, at the time of his colleague's death, was being investigated for alleged misuse of regimental funds.

The military court convened to consider the circumstances of Watters's death, returned a verdict of suicide by hanging. With the enquiry concluded, Emmett-Dunne resumed his normal duties and, in the spring of 1954, he was posted back to Britain. In June of that year, he married Watters's widow. The provost authori-ties in Germany were already dubious about the inquest verdict and news of

Emmett-Dunne's marriage and possible motive for wanting to be rid of his rival reinforced doubts.

This reconsideration led to a decision to exhume Watters's body and carry out a second post-mortem. Consequently, in February 1955, Francis Camps found himself on an aircraft heading for Germany to supervise the exhumation at Cologne Military Cemetery. He concluded that the injuries to the neck were not the result of hanging but were caused by a blow delivered sideways at the throat, such as a karate chop. The blow broke the thyroid cartilage and was the cause of death. Tests were carried out at the British Military Hospital at Hostert to establish the degree of force needed to break a human larynx. Murder now looked a more likely prospect than suicide and Emmett-Dunne was arrested on 20 April 1955 and sent back to Germany to face a court-martial.

The tall, powerfully built Sergeant gave a fanciful account of a disagreement between himself and Reginald Watters while they were sat in his car. He claimed that his erstwhile friend was angry about what he regarded as his over-friendly relationship with his wife and threatened him with a gun. Believing Watters intended to kill him before taking his own life, Emmett-Dunne hit out in self-defence. When he man-handled Watters out of the car, he realised he had killed him and decided to string up his body in a fake suicide.

The court-martial lasted nine days, during which Camps gave evidence and attended a reconstruction of the crucial incident which was supposed to have taken place in the car. Emmett-Dunne, with the help of a volunteer playing the part of Sergeant Watters, demonstrated the way in which he claimed to have struck his fellow soldier. Camps observed this re-enactment with a critical eye. He knew that the injuries resulting from the blow demonstrated by Emmett-Dunne would have landed on the side of the neck, whereas the fatal blow had been directed at the throat. It seemed that Emmett-Dunne, who was known to have undergone commando training in 1942, felled Watters with a chop to the throat delivered with the side of the hand.

Returning to the courtroom, armed with diagrams showing the anatomy of the neck and with the dead man's larynx mounted in a transparent box, Francis Camps continued his evidence. He described what had happened as, '. . . straightforward mechanics'. Asked if death had resulted from hanging, he replied simply, 'No.' He said that the injuries carefully described by the army pathologist were consistent with the body being suspended after death. The court-martial concluded with a guilty verdict and Emmett-Dunne was sentenced to death. He was spared the gallows, though, because Britain had signed a convention with Germany whereby the death penalty would not be acted upon in crimes committed by British military personnel. A sentence of life imprisonment was imposed, of which the ex-Sergeant served ten years before being released in 1965.

In the wake of this affair, Francis Camps was appointed Honorary Consultant Pathologist to the British Army. He had shown the value of experimentation in the Emmett-Dunne case by arranging with a Japanese ju-jitsu expert to show him how a traditional martial arts blow would be delivered and with what amount of force. The purpose of this improvisation was to judge the difference between the way in which certain unarmed combat blows were delivered. He judged that the position and direction of a ju-jitsu blow was inconsistent with the injury that killed Sergeant Watters, whereas a commando-style chop would have delivered sufficient deadly force.

Christmas Humphreys, who appeared as prosecuting counsel in many murder trials, including that of Donald Hume, had numerous encounters with Francis Camps. In his autobiography, Humphreys referred to the pathologist in his index, perhaps mischievously, but certainly erroneously, as, 'Sir Francis', and went on to criticise him for occasionally answering first and thinking afterwards. He did, though, praise him as a pioneer in experimentation, what he called, 'practical pathology'. Camps himself looked upon experimentation as a valuable means of avoiding worn-out theories. The astute lawyer perhaps recognised an impetuosity in Camps's character that was not always his best quality.

Sir Arthur Conan Doyle observed, through comments attributed to Sherlock Holmes, that when a doctor goes wrong he is the 'first of criminal minds' because he has both nerve and knowledge. This seemed to apply to Dr John Bodkin Adams when he was charged with murder in 1956. Several of his patients died in suspicious circumstances after leaving him substantial legacies. Rumours had swirled around the general practitioner in his hometown, Eastbourne on the Sussex coast, for several years. These grew in intensity as his name frequently appeared as a beneficiary in the wills of his deceased patients, many of whom were elderly, wealthy widows. To all intents and purposes, he was an upright citizen and a servant of the community. He had practised in Eastbourne for over thirty years and lived the life of a bachelor. He had some 2,000 patients on his list, many of whom paid privately for his services.

Dr Adams had the good fortune to be left legacies by many of his grateful patients. A thousand pounds here, a few hundred there, enabling him to live comfortably, looked after by a housekeeper and employing a chauffeur. Undercurrents of gossip had begun to circulate in 1935 when a patient died and left him £3,000. A drip-feed of innuendo and knowing looks persisted for the next twenty years. Matters came to a head in July 1956 following the death of fifty-year-old Gertrude Hullett. She had been treated by Dr Adams, who prescribed barbiturate sleeping pills. The doctor drew suspicion to himself by writing to the coroner about what he termed a 'very peculiar case', and seeking to make arrangements for a private post-mortem for his patient, who was not yet dead. The coroner was surprised and, no doubt, shocked when he learned later that Adams had been left money and a Rolls-Royce by Mrs Hullett.

The lady died on 23 July and Dr Adams certified death as due to cerebral haem-orrhage. A post-mortem was ordered and Francis Camps found that Mrs Hullett had taken a fatal dose of barbiturates, amounting to 115 grains. The coroner's inquest returned a verdict of suicide and Dr Adams came in for some sharp criti-cism from the coroner who reprimanded him for 'careless treatment'. The press seized on the suspicions building up around the Eastbourne doctor and all but accused him of murder. Deaths of his patients over the preceding twenty years were brought into view and speculation was rife. The police had been carrying out enquiries and taken an interest in the death in 1950 of eighty-one-year-old Edith Morrell. Dr Adams had been treating her for arthritis with heroin and morphine to relieve the pain. In her gratitude, she bequeathed her car and some silver cutlery to her doctor. When he was informed of the public interest in Mrs Morrell's death, Dr Adams said, 'Easing the passing of a dying patient is not all that wicked. She wanted to die. That cannot be murder.' On 19 December 1956, Dr Adams was arrested and charged with murdering Edith Morrell.

The police had applied for exhumation orders in respect of two former patients who had died while under the doctor's care. He sought help from the Medical Defence Union who asked Dr Keith Simpson to maintain a watching brief as far as the exhumations were concerned. In the event, only one body offered any prospect of a useful autopsy and Camps and Simpson agreed that cerebral throm-bosis was the cause of death which confirmed what Dr Adams had recorded at the time. From the investigators' point of view, it was a pity that the murder charge was brought in connection with Mrs Morrell's death. The fact that she had been cremated made the prosecution's task more difficult. Crucial evidence at Dr Adams's trial at the Old Bailey was given by the nurses who had attended the old lady. Their recollections of what had taken place six years previously appeared to be at variance with notes made in the nursing logbooks.

The outcome of the trial was generally regarded as a triumph for Geoffrey Lawrence QC who exploited weaknesses in the prosecution's case. His ruthless cross-examination of Dr Arthur Douthwaite, a colleague of Keith Simpson's at Guy's, was pivotal to the proceedings. The doctor said there was no justifica-tion for administering barbiturates to patients following a stroke and his evidence unequivocally pointed the finger at Dr Adams whose intention in prescribing drugs for Mrs Morrell was 'to terminate her life'. But counsel was able to show from her medical records that four doctors had seen her on different occasions and all had prescribed morphia. He also pointed out that Dr Adams had made fewer visits to his patient and administered less morphia than was supposed. Keith Simpson's view was that 'subtle pressure' had been put on Dr Douthwaite to give his testimony against Adams, who declined to take the witness stand.

This meant that evidence relating to patients other than Mrs Morrell was not permitted. Hence it was not possible for the nurse in attendance on one of them to repeat what she had said at the time:'You realise, Doctor, that you have killed her.'

Francis Camps was called to give evidence on the thirteenth day of what, at that time, was the longest murder trial conducted in Britain. He was asked by the Attorney-General, Sir Reginald Manningham-Buller, to deal with questions related to cremation and the role of a second doctor or medical referee. The pathologist outlined the procedure which required two doctors to sign a form authorising cremation. He said that where the deceased had expressed a wish to be cremated, it had become the practice to carry out a post-mortem because, as he very succinctly phrased it, 'cremation is the final act'. Asked about the feelings relatives might have regarding the need for post-mortems, Camps gave a careful reply to the effect that in circumstances where relatives might prefer burial in full knowledge that a deceased person had made a bequest in favour of the attending doctor, the medical referee, or second doctor, would automatically notify the coroner. His comments would have resonance forty years later when another medical practitioner, Dr Harold Shipman, was tried for murder.

On 10 April 1957, Dr Adams was found not guilty. He resigned from the National Health Service, although he continued to live in Eastbourne. He was struck off the Medical Register and there was public disquiet when the Director of Public Prosecutions declined to proceed against the doctor with other accusations of murder. Many believed that Adams murdered for gain, while other, more charitable commentators, suggested he simply practised euthanasia. The doctor regained his medical registration in 1961 and resumed his practice in Eastbourne where he died, aged eighty-four, in 1983.

Dr Adams certainly benefited from his years of medical practice. At the time of his death, his estate was valued at over £400,000 and he earned £10,000 from a national newspaper for his life story. A sale of his possessions raised £12,000 and the doctor's medical bag bearing his initials went for £92. Unusually in a murder case, the trial judge, Patrick Devlin, wrote a book about it, called *Easing the Passing*, published in 1985. He retired early, reportedly because he found his work tedious, and died in 1992.

Francis Camps had been appointed Reader in Forensic Medicine at the London Hospital in 1954 and two years later collaborated with his friend, Bentley Purchase, to produce a textbook, *Practical Forensic Medicine*. Described as 'the most famous coroner of his day', Purchase began his career in the late 1950s and shared Camps's no nonsense approach to their work. This joint effort was the first indication of their determination to put forensic investigation on the map and was a springboard for greater things to come.

According to his biographer, Robert Jackson, Camps was not a particularly effective lecturer. He tended to be over-enthusiastic and was easily blown off course by minor diversions. He did, though, have what observers described as a wicked sense of humour and was not always popular with his students. On one occasion in 1963 when he spoke to undergraduate members of the Chemical Society at Southampton University, it was apparent that he had not prepared too well. He brought with him a hastily assembled collection of projection slides which he used as prompts for a rambling account of practical forensic medicine. Unsurprisingly, many of his illustrations were of partially dissected or decomposing corpses on the mortuary table. This had a startling effect on some unsuspecting members of his audience who fainted in their seats or made a dash for the exit. Calls were put out to the St John's Ambulance for assistance. While he was, possibly, not the most gifted of lecturers, Francis Camps compensated with his organisational and writing skills.

Meanwhile, routine forensic investigations proceeded apace and he frequently found himself in opposition to Keith Simpson. This was so in a case which captured headlines in July 1955 with the death of five-month-old Terence, the son of John and Janet Armstrong. It was supposed that the boy had eaten poisonous berries from the garden given to him innocently by his three-year-old sister who had also eaten some. She was sick but otherwise not ill.

A post-mortem carried out on Terence showed the presence in his stomach and trachea of red skins, presumed to be remnants of the berries. The doctor was not able to give a cause of death and the inquest into the boy's death was opened and then adjourned. The parents were interviewed by the police and officers were surprised by the apparent lack of grief. Twenty-five-year-old John Armstrong, a Navy Sick Bay Attendant at the Royal Naval Hospital at Haslar in Portsmouth, lived with his twenty-year-old wife, Janet, and their two young children at Gosport. Detectives had their suspicions that the cause of death was not the berries and arranged for the skins retrieved from the child's body to be sent to Scotland Yard's Forensic Laboratory. Tests showed that there was a significant quantity of the drug, Seconal, in the sample. The supposed red berry skins were in fact the gelatine coating of Seconal capsules. Dr Lewis Nickolls, chief scientist at the laboratory, estimated the child had consumed about five Seconal capsules. The drug was a powerful barbiturate normally prescribed to assist sleeping.

The Armstrong family now came under scrutiny and it was discovered that the couple's first son had died in 1954 from broncho-pneumonia. Their home at Gosport was searched with no suspicious consequences. Meanwhile, authority had been given for Terence Armstrong's body to be exhumed. Keith Simpson conducted the post-mortem examination and concluded that the boy had died of a massive overdose of Seconal. Detectives checking on John Armstrong and his duties at Haslar Naval Hospital found that a cupboard containing dangerous drugs had been broken into several months previously and, among the items missing, were Seconal capsules.

On 1 September 1956, over a year after Terence Armstrong's death, his parents were arrested and charged with murder. By this time, Mr and Mrs Armstrong had separated and Janet admitted there was Seconal in the house which her husband took to help him sleep. On his instructions she had disposed of the remaining capsules. The Armstrongs were committed for trial at Winchester when Norman Skelhorn, a future Director of Public Prosecutions, appeared on behalf of Janet, and Francis Camps was retained to assist the defence.

John Armstrong denied all knowledge of how his son was poisoned. Janet said that he had the opportunity when he returned home for lunch on the fatal day, to be alone with his son. She also confirmed that there had been Seconal in the house. Each party blamed the other in a 'cut-throat' defence. The jury found John Armstrong guilty while Janet was acquitted. The death sentence imposed on John was reduced to life imprisonment and, a month after the trial concluded, his wife admitted, via the pages of a Sunday newspaper, that she had given her son one capsule of Seconal to help him sleep. In his autobiography, Keith Simpson recorded his pleasure at not being 'bested by Camps', as he put it, and recorded that three years later, 'the boot was on the other foot' when he assisted in the defence of Sergeant Marcus Marymont, and Camps helped the prosecution. Simpson, at least, appeared to relish his adversarial contests with Francis Camps.

Two cases involving poisonous elements – phosphorus in one, and arsenic in the other – commanded Camps's involvement in 1958. While arsenic had, for centuries, been a favourite lethal agent used by poisoners, phosphorus poisoning is relatively uncommon. Mary Wilson lived in County Durham in the delightfully named district of Windy Nook. Four men in her life who she took as either husbands or lovers died in suspicious circumstances and earned her the title of 'The Poisoner of Windy Nook'. Sixty-six-year-old Mary was an unprepossessing woman with red hair and, from all accounts, a person with a mean streak. She also harboured a passion for romance. Her early life was spent in service to a family in the industrial north east of England. She married the son of her employers and, when he died, she switched her attentions to the man who lodged at the house. He also died soon afterwards. Few questions were asked about the deaths of two elderly men in the same house and the local doctor believed they had both died of natural causes.

In 1957, Mary met Oliver James Leonard, an elderly retired estate agent of modest means, who lived in lodgings. They married in September but Leonard fell ill with a severe cold and died two weeks later. He had consulted a doctor because he was feeling unwell and a death certificate was issued as a matter of course. Mary Wilson benefited from her late husband's estate to the tune of £50, which was all the money he possessed. Her next move was to respond to an elderly retired engineer who was looking for a housekeeper. She went to live with him and they were soon married. Ernest Wilson, Mary's new husband, became ill through eating liver, or so she said when she sent for the doctor. The next day, two weeks after they had married, Ernest died. Death was certified as due to heart failure.

Far from playing the role of a grieving widow, Mary indulged in black humour, suggesting to the undertaker that he quote her a wholesale price for a coffin. As rumours began to circulate, she told acquaintances, 'I didn't mean to kill them. They were dead already.' This was presumably a reference to the fact that they were all elderly men. By raising the stakes against herself with unwise utterances, Mary Wilson soon found herself talking to the police. As in the case of Dr Bodkin Adams, the circulation of rumours can be the springboard for enquiries in cases of suspected poisoning.

The bodies of Oliver Leonard and Ernest Wilson were exhumed and post-mortems showed that their deaths were certainly not due to natural causes. In both instances, lethal quantities of phosphorus were found. It was noted that Mary Wilson had attempted to deflect suspicion from herself by asking doctors to examine her husbands prior to their deaths. The suggestion was that phosphorus, probably in the form of powdered beetle killer, had been administered in doses of cough mixture.

Mary Wilson was sent for trial at Leeds Assizes and Francis Camps was briefed for the defence. Supported by four expert witnesses, the prosecution's case was that both husbands had died of first-stage phosphorus poisoning. The amounts of poison found at post-mortem indicated that relatively large doses were involved. Defence counsel, Rose Heilbron QC, introduced what she described as a novel diversion when she suggested that Mary Wilson's husbands might have taken aphrodisiac pills containing phosphorus. Such a sexual stimulant was apparently available over the counter for public use. This suggestion inevitably produced laughter in court but the prosecution countered it by saying each of the victims would have had to consume 150 such pills to account for the levels of phosphorus found in their bodies.

The evidence given by Francis Camps was not based on having examined the victims but on his understanding of the medical reports. Whereas the prosecution experts had theoretical knowledge of phosphorus poisoning, Camps had direct experience. He was extremely circumspect in the opinions he gave, to the extent that his biographer wondered whether it was worthwhile for him to have travelled north. Asked if he would give a cause of death, the pathologist said he believed the post-mortem findings were contradictory and he pointed out the absence of microscopical evidence. On that basis be declined to give an opinion, saying simply, that cause of death was 'unascertainable'. His reasoning was that other possible causes had not been eliminated. On the face of it, his views seemed to be critical of the experts aiding the prosecution. He also strongly made the point that no autopsy in any case of poisoning could be considered complete without full pathological examination of the relevant adjoining organs.

Francis Camps's careful perspective of phosphorus poisoning did not particularly help the defence and Mary Wilson was found guilty of murder. She was sentenced to death but secured a reprieve, as noted in *A Calendar of Murder*, '. . . presumably because she was an old woman'. The 'Poisoner of Windy Nook', who murdered four times for the modest gain of £200, was sentenced to life imprisonment. She died in prison at the age of seventy. Her tally of victims increased as the result of inquests held on the two men she had lived with earlier in her life. In both cases, phosphorus poisoning was recorded. As a footnote, it is worth mentioning Sir Sydney Smith's comment about phosphorus poisoning which he said declined with the demise of yellow-tipped matches.

The trial of the 'Poisoner of Windy Nook' highlighted some of the deficiencies in the system of presenting forensic evidence in court. Camps was already resolved through his teaching programme at the London Hospital to raise standards, and in 1958 took a huge step forward by setting up the British Academy of Forensic Sciences (BAFS). He did this in association with his friend, the solicitor Sir David Napley. In his memoir, *Not Without Prejudice*, Napley described their objective which was to overcome the virtual absence of 'any knowledge of forensic medicine among lawyers and an inadequate level of knowledge among the medical profession'. Francis Camps had been influenced by the work of the American Academy of Forensic Sciences which he had seen at first hand during his visits to the USA. To add to his already busy schedule, he now became Secretary of BAFS.

In the summer of 1958, Camps was able to indulge his inclination for experimentation in a case of arsenic poisoning. Not for the first time he found himself dealing with the misdemeanours of a serviceman with the rank of Sergeant. Thirty-seven-year-old Master Sergeant Marcus Marymont of the United States Air Force, was based at Sculthorpe in Norfolk, an airfield from which secret reconnaissance flights operated during the Cold War. Marymont lived in married quarters with his wife, Mary Helen, and their three children. They had been in Britain for over two years. The marriage had run into difficulties and Marymont became increasingly attracted by the nightlife of London. He spent a large proportion of his off-duty time away from home, while Mary Helen was left on her own, believing her husband's absence was due to assignment on temporary duties. In July 1956, at a pub near Maidenhead, the Master Sergeant met twenty-year-old Cynthia Taylor who had separated from her husband after four months of marriage. They danced and were attracted to each other.

As the relationship developed, Marymont explained to his girlfriend that he was divorced and his ex-wife lived in America. He and Cynthia talked about marrying when her own divorce was finalised. On 8 June 1958, the Marymonts were invited out to lunch with friends. Mary Helen looked unwell and she and her husband left early. On the following day, she was admitted to hospital at the

USAF base, suffering with gastric problems. Her condition worsened, and when she lapsed into unconsciousness, there were fears for her life. The anxieties were well founded for she did not respond to emergency measures and died in hospital. The base doctor noted that Marymont appeared to be remarkably unmoved by his wife's death. He gave permission for an autopsy to be carried out to determine the cause of Mary Helen's death. Then, he attempted to withdraw his consent but was overruled by the military authorities who insisted that a post-mortem was necessary.

Francis Camps was called on in his capacity as a Home Office pathologist and set about removing organs from the dead woman's body for laboratory analysis. Critically, he also took samples of hair. Dr Lewis Nickolls of the Metropolitan Police Laboratory, carried out tests that showed traces of arsenic in the liver which were indicative of a poisonous dose having been ingested twenty-four hours prior to death. Human hair has an absorbent capacity which makes its examination particularly important in cases of poisoning. Poison is picked up from the bloodstream and drawn into the hair, creating a marker which enables an analyst to work out the approximate strength and frequency of dosage. By these means, Dr Nickolls was able to ascertain that Mary Helen Marymont had absorbed doses of arsenic over a period of about six months.

Enquiries into the source of the arsenic centered on Marcus Marymont's attempt to buy some from a pharmacy in Maidenhead. He did not persist with his request when told he needed to provide some documentation. He was more successful when he visited the laboratory at the USAF base where he was stationed. His request met with a favourable response, which led him to quip with staff that bottles containing arsenic should be kept under lock and key. His humour turned somewhat sour when he was arrested and charged with murdering his wife with poison.

While the Master Sergeant awaited his appearance at a court-martial, Francis Camps exercised his talent for experimentation. He wanted to determine how arsenic might be administered. He learned that, taken by mouth, or even in food, arsenic causes a strong burning sensation which is immediately apparent. Whereas, a strong dose of 10 grains or more could be disguised in, for example, coffee or cocoa, without causing an objectionable taste. He survived to relate his experiences so, presumably, he did not swallow his test beverages.

Marymont's court-martial was convened at Denham in Buckinghamshire in September 1958. The proceedings were conducted under American jurisdiction, which included a panel of officers acting as judges. The prosecution argued simply that the Master Sergeant wanted his wife out of the way so that he would be free to marry his lover. He tried to poison her with small doses of arsenic and when that failed to have the desired effect, he resorted to a heavy dose with fatal consequences. The defendant maintained his innocence and suggested that his wife's illness was caused by self-administered arsenic in an attempt to win back his affections. Defence counsel claimed the evidence against Marymont was circumstantial. Cynthia Taylor underwent the ordeal of being on the witness stand for over six hours, during which, letters that had passed between her and Marymont were read out. This had the effect of exposing the lies he had told her about his marital status.

When Francis Camps was called to give evidence, it was apparent that those administering the court-martial procedure had little knowledge as to the depth of his experience. His response to counsel's question about the number of post-mortems he had carried out created a minor sensation. His answer, that he thought the number was around 60,000 produced sharp intakes of breath on the part of many present. He dealt with issues of how arsenic might have been administered without Mrs Marymont realising it and dismissed the notion that her death was suicide. He observed, knowingly, that people who took poison to gain sympathy were only too anxious to go on living. The military judges deliberated for over five hours before finding Marymont guilty on two charges of murder and adultery. He was sentenced to life imprisonment with hard labour and dishonourably discharged from the US Air Force. He lost his subsequent appeal, although the adultery charge was dropped, and he was returned to the USA to serve his sentence at Fort Leavenworth Prison in Kansas.

At the height of his powers, Francis Camps was conducting around fifty post-mortems a week. He, and his friend, Sir Bentley Purchase, coroner for the northern district of London, dominated the forensic map in their area. Camps was a pioneering pathologist and he used his fame to make professional advances, not for personal aggrandisement, but to enhance the status of forensic investigation. He built up state-of-the-art facilities at the London Hospital which became his operational base. Part of his ambition, which he shared with Bentley Purchase and David Napley, was to harness all the advantages of science to aid the forensic pathologist. By the late 1950s, he had gathered around him a team of specialists whose skills embraced serology, chemistry, dentistry and medical photography to complement the core discipline of forensic medicine.

Woven into all the run-of-the-mill cases which came his way, there were always the weird and unusual episodes. None was more curious than the 'Mummy of Rhyl'. Sarah Jane Harvey, a widow aged sixty-five, lived in the seaside town of Rhyl in North Wales. She occasionally took in paying guests. In May 1960, Mrs Harvey was admitted to hospital for tests. While she was away, her son, Leslie, decided to freshen up the interior of her house with some painting and decorating.

On the landing at the top of the stairs was a large wooden cupboard which Mrs Harvey always kept locked. Leslie decided to open it but, in light of what he found, perhaps wished he had not. Inside was a dried-out corpse festooned in cobwebs, dirt and dead flies. The local doctor viewed the body and thought a forensic specialist was required. Dr Gerald Evans, a Home Office pathologist based at Bangor, was called to the scene. He was confronted by a set of human remains that had been transformed into a granite-hard shell of skin and bone. Clearly, the body had been in place for some considerable time. It was so firmly stuck to the floor of the cupboard that a garden spade had to be used to prise it loose. Dr Evans had the body removed to the mortuary where initial examination indicated the remains were those of a middle-aged woman. X-rays showed no signs of fractures or the presence of any foreign objects. The body was placed in a bath of dilute glycerine to soften the tissues and permit examination of the internal organs. The pathologist traced a groove in the neck in which lay the remains of a cloth ligature. The age of the body was estimated at between forty and sixty.

The discovery at her home prompted a visit to Mrs Harvey from the police. She had an interesting story to tell. During the early weeks of the Second World War, that is, in 1939, she provided board and lodgings for a lady called Frances Knight, who was a semi-invalid. A few weeks later, she found Mrs Knight complaining of severe pain which resulted in her collapse and death. In this unexpected situation, Mrs Harvey decided the best course of action was to say nothing and hide the body. So, she dragged the dead woman along the upstairs landing and pushed her into the cupboard which she firmly locked. And there it remained for twenty years until its chance discovery by her son. During this time, Mrs Harvey continued to collect weekly rent which was paid by her late boarder's estranged husband.

Enquiries established that Frances Knight had attended a hospital in Liverpool in 1939 and been diagnosed with disseminated sclerosis. The extraordinary condition of her body when discovered was popularly described as mummification; after all, 'The Mummy of Rhyl' made a good headline. The remains had become dessicated as part of a natural process accompanied by air movements in and around the cupboard. Cause of death was not immediately apparent but attention focussed on the ligature around her neck and discussion of whether, or not, it had contributed to Mrs Knight's death.

A prosecution for murder was brought against Sarah Harvey and she appeared for trial at Ruthin Assizes in October 1960. Dr Evans was the expert witness for the prosecution while Francis Camps and the redoubtable Sydney Smith advised the defence team. A successful prosecution depended on the interpretation placed on the remains of a knotted stocking found around the neck of the mummified body. Dr Evans was thorough in his presentation of the facts and said that the actual cause of death was unascertainable. He was not able to say whether the ligature had been placed around the neck before or after death. The localised deep groove in the skin suggested that the ligature had been tight.

Although present in court, neither Camps nor Smith was called upon to give direct evidence. Defence counsel, briefed by the two pathologists, cast doubt on the ligature as a means of strangulation. The suggestion was made that the stocking around the neck might have a simple and innocent explanation. Mention was made of the custom in the North of England to tie a sock around a person who was ill as a kind of comfort. Camps noted that this suggestion met with nods of understanding among some of those in the courtroom. The defence was also able to show that Mrs Knight's illness could have resulted in death from natural causes.

On the fifth day of the trial, prosecuting counsel, Sir Jocelyn Simon, told the court that he believed if would be unsafe to pursue the murder charge. The judge agreed and Sarah Harvey was found not guilty, although she was convicted on a charge of obtaining money by false pretences. She was sentenced to fifteen months' imprisonment for this misdemeanour. Harvey had maintained her deception for twenty years, leading people to believe that Mrs Knight was still alive and benefiting to the tune of more than £2,000.

Francis Camps was criticised by some for being overbearing at times and lacking in generosity towards colleagues. But, he clearly admired the work carried out by the Welsh pathologist, Gerald Evans, on the mummified remains. In his book, *Camps on Crime*, published the year after his death, he devoted a chapter to 'The Mummy of Rhyl' which carried an account by Gerald Evans on the pathological investigation he had carried out. Camps particularly noted, 'the meticulous care taken by Dr Evans' and acknowledged that 'much useful scientific knowledge had been acquired'.

Camps notched up a hat-trick of cases involving servicemen with the rank of Sergeant when he gave evidence at the Boshears trial in 1961. This centred on a controversial death by strangulation which had distant echoes of the Chrissie Gall case in 1932 when the evidence of Spilsbury and Smith favouring suicide was disregarded by the jury which opted instead for murder. While self-strangulation was uncommon; a strangler killing in his sleep was even rarer.

Staff Sergeant Willis Eugene Boshears, a twenty-nine-year-old married serviceman in the US Air Force, was based at Wetherfield in Essex. On New Year's Eve 1960, Boshears was alone at his flat in Dunmow, while his wife and children were staying with her parents. Fed up with being on his own, he decided to visit some of the local pubs where he embarked on a drinking spree, which included consuming vodka, whisky and beer. At The Bell in Braintree, he met twenty-year-old Jean Constable who was in the pub with a man friend. She was a regular in the local pubs and was drawn to the US servicemen who had money to spend and were out for a good time. She and her friend joined Boshears in dancing to music played on the jukebox and, then he invited the couple back to his flat where more drinking and jiving ensued.

Sensing that his guests were intent on having sex, Boshears showed them into the bedroom and left them to it. Later, he pulled a mattress in front of the fire and all three lay down together. Jean Constable went to sleep and, around 1 a.m., her companion decided to leave. By this time, Boshears had passed out after his long session of binge drinking. What happened next was described by Boshears after Constable's body was discovered in a water-filled ditch in the Essex countryside. He remembered laying down beside the girl who was already asleep and then he passed out. The next thing he recalled was something scratching at his face. He woke up and found Constable lying beneath him. He had his hand on her throat and realised that she was dead.

In a state of panic, he cut off the dead girl's hair to make identification difficult, tidied up the flat and put her body in the spare room while he decided what to do. Two days later, he drove out into the countryside and dumped the body in a ditch where it was discovered by a passing lorry driver. It was not long before the police became aware of how Jean Constable had spent an evening drinking and jiving with a Sergeant from the USAAF base. Boshears was arrested and charged with murder. The US authorities wanted to try him by court-martial, against the wishes of the Essex Police. The Director of Public Prosecutions upheld the police view that Boshears should be judged in a British court and, so, he was tried at Essex Assizes in Chelmsford in February 1961.

Francis Camps had conducted the post-mortem examination of Jean Constable's body and concluded that her death was caused by asphyxia resulting from manual strangulation. He thought pressure had been applied to the throat for about thirty seconds. In court, Boshears pleaded not guilty to murder. He made many denials; there had been no arguments, no quarrels, no sexual advances and no wish to harm the young woman. Reminded by the prosecutor that he had attempted to cover up the crime, Boshears accepted that he had done so. Asked what crime he thought he had committed, he answered, 'The logical one.' Invited to expand on his answer, he said, 'I had killed someone.'

In giving his evidence, Francis Camps attempted to reconstruct the sequence of events which had overwhelmed Jean Constable. He said she would have resisted pressure on her throat, even if involuntarily. He made the point that everyone unconsciously protects themselves. Then she would have lapsed into uncon-sciousness followed by convulsion and death. He believed this process might have taken half a minute. The pathologist's first conclusion was that the idea of a man strangling a woman in his sleep sounded improbable. But, he later modified this opinion by saying he did not think it was impossible.

In his summing up, Mr Justice Glyn-Jones advised the jury to apply common sense. 'Have you ever heard of a man strangling a woman while he was sound asleep?' he asked, although he reminded them that Dr Camps had said it might be possible. Camps did not share the learned judge's sense of incredulity because he probably knew that in 1952, a consultant psychiatrist giving evidence at a criminal trial in Devon had commented that somnambulistic attacks were not uncommon. On that occasion, a naval officer had been acquitted of attempted murder while sleepwalking. And, in 1943, a teenage girl in Kentucky, USA, had been acquitted of a charge of murdering her father and brother while sleepwalking.

The jury returned a not guilty verdict in the case of Sergeant Boshears and he walked from the courtroom into a barrage of public indignation. Many who had gathered to hear news of the verdict were shocked at the acquittal, while Boshears expressed his appreciation of British justice. Five months later, he returned to the USA where he was subsequently dismissed from the Air Force. Robert Jackson, in his biography of Camps, noted the pathologist's wry observation that it was rare for a defence based on accidental death to succeed in a case where a body had been concealed.

Camps had, again, demonstrated his measured approach, balancing doubts and probabilities and eschewing the cut-and-dried opinions for which Spilsbury was famous. As subsequent events would show, keeping an open mind was crucial to the whole forensic process. In 1992, for example, a man whose identity was protected by law was acquitted at Newcastle Crown Court on a charge of attempted murder. He had, apparently, tried to strangle his teenage son while sleepwalking. He was judged to have been suffering from insane automatism at the time of the incident. And in 2009, a man was cleared of murder at Swansea Crown Court after he strangled his wife during a nightmare. He had a history of sleep disorders and suffered from a condition termed *pavor nocturnus*. The background was that he dreamt someone had broken into his accommodation while he was asleep and he attacked his wife believing she was the intruder.

Francis Camps was appointed Professor of Forensic Medicine in the University of London at the London Hospital Medical School in 1963. He continued to build up his department as a widely recognised centre of excellence and he undertook lectures at numerous London medical schools, including the Middlesex, Royal Free and University College. He also devoted a great deal of time and energy to the British Academy of Forensic Sciences, to which he had been appointed Secretary in 1958, and edited the BAFS journal, *Medicine, Science and the Law*. Through the publicity which he attracted with his involvement in high-profile murder cases, he had also become a public figure or what, today, would be deemed a celebrity. His photograph frequently appeared in the popular press, always immaculately dressed, invariably smoking a pipe and looking very professional.

One of his many gifts, commented on by Sir David Napley, was that Camps always knew the right people. Thus, he had persuaded Professor Leon Radzinowitz, Director of the Institute of Criminology at Cambridge University, to become the first President of BAFS and he lured several medico-legal luminaries of the day to join his editorial board, including Lord Birkett and Sir Frederick Lawton, both eminent judges, and two fellow pathologists, Dr Donald Teare and Professor John Glaister. By virtue of his persuasive personality, he had succeeded in drawing together exemplars from the fields of medicine, science and the law into a common enterprise.

Napley was Chairman of the Executive Council of BAFS and in his memoir, *Not Without Prejudice*, he wrote that his most difficult task was to confront Francis Camps. He said, 'It was like harnessing a meteor.' His thought processes did not flow along accustomed lines and he tended to flit from one subject to another. Among his friend's weaknesses, Napley mentioned Camps's dislike of Keith Simpson and his fear of contracting cancer. For a man with a medical background who smoked cigarettes and a pipe, this must have been a real concern. After his old friend and mentor, seventy-year-old Sir Bentley Purchase, died unexpectedly, following an accident at his home in September 1961, Camps might have felt the pull of mortality. If he did, it was not noticeable for he continued to work at the same relentless pace, devoting much of his time and energy to writing.

In April 1966, he published an article in *The London Hospital Gazette* on the subject of Jack the Ripper, the unknown perpetrator of the Whitechapel Murders in 1888. His assistant, 'Sam' Hardy, had discovered in London Hospital's archives hitherto unpublicised letters, sketches and scene-of-crime maps relating to the murders. Of particular interest were pencil sketches made at the murder scene by Dr F. Gordon Brown, City of London Police Surgeon, of the wounds inflicted on Catherine Eddowes who was murdered in Mitre Square. If anyone could shed light on a subject that had been plagued with all kinds of nonsense over the years, surely it was Francis Camps.

In an interview with *Medical News*, he gave it as his opinion that the real cause of death in Jack the Ripper's victims was strangulation, rather than the throat-cutting which followed. He pointed out that contemporary reports in *The Lancet* mentioned that the faces of the victims were congested which, he suggested, accounted for the fact that they did not cry out. Camps found nothing in these new discoveries to support the notion that the Whitechapel Murderer had any anatomical skill or, indeed, any association with the London Hospital, either as a student or a doctor.

The discovery of these documents caused a flurry of excitement in the media. Never one to shy away from publicity, Camps and his colleagues at the London Hospital gave interviews to the major newspapers and they were overwhelmed with inquiries from writers and researchers interested in these historic crimes. In October 1966, he continued his interest in the Ripper murders by taking what he called a 'new look' at them in his book, *The Investigation of Murder*, co-written with Richard Barber. The first part of the book was devoted to headline murder cases, including Maybrick, Crippen and Christie and a look at the development of scientific methods of investigation. The main thrust of the book, though, was to explore the management of forensic work in the future. He stressed the importance of organisation and wrote about the requirements for education, training and research. He singled out teamwork as the most vital factor in strengthening the relationship between forensic science and forensic medicine. An appendix to his text consisted of a diagram showing how all the elements could be brought together within a university framework to serve the needs of the police and the law courts. It was a model of a kind of forensic utopia.

During his visits to the USA in the 1950s, Camps met Dr Rutherford Gradwohl, a distinguished forensic expert, who modernised the US approach to medical examination. He and Camps shared the ideal of bringing medicine and science together, and Gradwohl's police laboratory which he set up in St Louis in 1954 was greatly admired. Gradwohl also edited an authoritative textbook on legal medicine and it was his wish that Francis Camps should succeed him as editor. The second edition of *Legal Medicine* was published under Camps's editorship in 1968, following his predecessor's death. The textbook won acclaim as an acknowledged and reliable source for doctors, lawyers and scientists by bringing together the elements of best practice from both sides of the Atlantic. In that respect alone, it reflected the ideals which Camps had pursued throughout his professional life. It was said that if Gradwohl was the father of legal medicine, then Camps was its mentor.

A controversial case in the Canadian courts brought Francis Camps into confrontation with his old adversary, Keith Simpson, in 1967. Some harsh words were spoken about Camps's performance but, in an ironic twist to the story over forty years later, the Mentor would be vindicated. In the summer of 1959, a murder in Ontario, involving two youngsters, Lynne Harper, aged twelve, and Steven Truscott, aged fourteen, victim and suspect, shocked Canada. On the evening of 9 June, Lynne left her home near Clinton and failed to return. A search for the missing girl located her body two days later in a wooded area called Lawson's Bush. She had been raped and strangled. The last sighting of her alive was between 7 and 7.45 on the evening that she disappeared.

The post-mortem was carried out by Dr John Penistan, Ontario's official pathologist. He found that the dead girl's stomach contained both digested and undigested food, consistent with the meal she had eaten with her parents at around 5.30 p.m. The pathologist determined that she had died within two hours of eating the meal. From the beginning of the investigation, attention focused on Steven Truscott. When questioned, he said he had met Lynne in order to give her a lift on his bike to a place a short distance away where there were some horses she wanted to see. A woman saw the pair leave together just before 7 p.m. Steven said he dropped Lynne off and then cycled back. He chatted with friends at the football field before returning home at around 8.25 p.m.

Steven was questioned several times. His replies were consistent and he mentioned that when he left her, he saw Lynne hitch a lift in a grey Chevrolet with a yellow number plate. He was subjected to a medical examination and doctors found a sore patch on his penis which they concluded had been the result of committing rape. Steven Truscott was charged with murder and his guilt was cut-and-dried as far as local opinion was concerned. His trial for murder took place in the adult court at Goderich, Ontario in September. The key prosecution evidence was given by Dr Penistan, supported by Dr David Brooks, a Royal Canadian Air Force physician, who had been present at the post-mortem on Lynne Harper. Referring to the dead girl's stomach contents, they confirmed their initial findings which put the girl's death between 7 and 7.45 p.m. and coincided exactly with the time that she had been seen with Truscott.

This interpretation was challenged by the defence expert, Dr Berkeley Brown, who told the court that the time taken to empty the stomach was longer than the estimates given by the prosecution. By his reckoning, the time of death would have been an hour later, at a time when Steven was known to have returned home. Reference was made to the sore on his penis and the doctor who had examined him testified that he believed it was consistent with committing rape. An alternative speculation was that it was due to an allergy.

The jury returned a guilty verdict with a plea for mercy. The judge sentenced Steven Truscott to death, the execution being scheduled for 8 December 1959. An appeal to the Supreme Court of Ontario failed and an application was made to appeal to the Supreme Court of Canada. This was also refused but sentence of death was commuted to life imprisonment. There matters rested until 1966 when the writer, Isabel Le Bourdais, published an account of the trial in which she strongly criticised the prosecution case. Her book, *The Trial of Steven Truscott*, carried a blunt question: 'Six years ago, at the age of fourteen, he was sentenced to death. Today, he is in the penitentiary at Kingston, Ontario. The question is: was he guilty?' The book and the issues it raised created considerable disquiet throughout Canada. As a result, pressure mounted for a re-examination of the case which took place in an unprecedented hearing before nine judges of the Supreme Court of Canada. The issue was to consider if there were any grounds for a retrial.

The publishers of Le Bourdais's book sent review copies to both Keith Simpson and Francis Camps. Simpson reviewed it for the *Medico-Legal Journal*, taking the view that the author's conclusions were biased and unfounded. Camps, on the other hand, adopted an opposing view which was that the medical evidence was not strong enough to support a conviction. The pace quickened and there was a flurry of excitement among the forensic medicine fraternities on both sides of the Atlantic. The result was that Simpson accepted an invitation from the Canadian Government to give evidence before the Supreme Court in Ottawa in support of the Crown's case, while Camps was invited to help the defence. He was aided by Dr Charles Petty, a pathologist based in Baltimore.

Also promoting the prosecution case was Dr Milton Helpern, the distinguished New York Medical Examiner. In his memoirs, *Autopsy*, written with Bernard Knight, he noted, '. . . we had seven forensic pathologists ready to argue the case.' It is in the nature of such high-level engagements that the professionals involved know each other, if not personally, then by reputation. Helpern described Francis Camps as, 'one of those restless, enthusiastic men who sometimes stampede down the wrong track'. Certainly, after reading the Le Bourdais book, Camps was voluble in his opinion that Truscott's conviction was not sustainable. In fact, he had, perhaps unwisely, written to the Attorney-General in England offering to give evidence in support of Truscott. Simpson leapt on this 'unethical offer of services', as he phrased it, and Camps was taken to task for it during the hearing in Ottawa.

The key issue remained that of determining when Lynne Harper had died. Dr Penistan, once again, presented his findings, supported by Helpern and Simpson. Their view was that Penistan was entirely correct in the conclusion he had reached in putting time of death in the narrow frame of 7 to 7.45 p.m. Dr Petty, backed by Camps, argued that it was not possible to make such a precise judgement from the state of the victim's stomach contents. They estimated that death had occurred in a much broader timeframe of one to ten hours. Max Haines, the noted Canadian crime reporter, summed up the prosecution medical evidence succinctly when he wrote, 'If the doctors were mistaken by a matter of an hour, Steven would have been in the company of other people and could not have been the killer.'

The outcome of the proceedings was that the judges decided there had been no miscarriage of justice and a re-trial was denied. Steven Truscott was returned to the penitentiary, where he remained until his release in 1969. Helpern criticised Francis Camps for being '. . . a somewhat incoherent speaker', whose 'brain raced ahead of his tongue'. Keith Simpson crowed that Camps had not 'come up to proof' and that '. . . the Crown and Dr Penistan had triumphed'. But, long after the main protagonists had died, the Truscott affair re-surfaced in the headlines in August 2007. Ontario's Supreme Court announced that Steven had been wrongfully convicted of rape and murder forty-eight years previously and cleared his name. It was ruled that post-mortem findings at the time allowed an estimate of time of death much later, perhaps a day later, than had been argued by the prosecution. This would have placed Truscott in the company of others and clearly lift suspicion from his shoulders. In 2008, he was awarded compensation amounting to £3.2 million.

Justice was served, although the murder of Lynne Harper remained unsolved. The Truscott case helped campaigners against the death penalty in Canada and the statute was abolished in 1976. The ironic reversal of forensic fortunes in this long and drawn-out affair in which Francis Camps's views had been derided at the time, gave him the last word. The eventual outcome went some way to endorse his philosophy that things are not always what they may seem.

Professor Camps was awarded the Swiney Prize in 1969 for his editorship of Gradwohl's *Legal Medicine*, described as the best publication in its field that year. He threw himself wholeheartedly into his teaching, giving lectures at three London hospitals and working as an examiner at five universities. His special contribution lay in his endeavours to break down the old barriers and put forensic studies on a modern footing. He led from the front, establishing a world class teaching department at the London Hospital and putting the British Academy of Forensic Sciences firmly on the map.

His retirement was blighted by bad feeling and poor health. Widely recognised as a man of affable personality, he also had a darker side which involved a strong dislike for some of his contemporaries, particularly Keith Simpson. His friend, David Napley, described the occasion in 1970 after Camps had announced his retirement and colleagues held a dinner in his honour in the City of London. Following a pleasant meal and with plaudits ringing in his ears, he rose to his feet with his friends expecting a warm and witty response to their good wishes. Instead, he launched into a bitter attack on some of his fellow pathologists and, without naming him, those present knew that much of his bile was directed at Keith Simpson. It was an uncomfortable moment and the evening finished on an embarrassing note.

There was a suggestion that he would use his time in retirement to write a biography of Sir Bernard Spilsbury. Doubtless, he would have put his own inimitable spin on the life of his predecessor but an admirable biography had been published in 1951 that was hardly likely to be bettered. When Camps experienced stomach pains, he convinced himself that he had cancer. Instead of seeking advice, he lived through the pain and tortured himself with the fear that when he died, it might fall to Keith Simpson to carry out the post-mortem. This was an irrational thought, as misplaced as his self-diagnosis. After he died on 8 July 1972, it was discovered that he had been suffering from stomach ulcers that could have been alleviated by surgery. It was a sad end for a man whose professional *raison d'être* was that appearances may conspire to deceive.

The death of Francis Camps resulted in fulsome tributes in the medical press. *The Lancet* referred to him as a '... marvellous tutor and mentor ...', while the *British Medical Journal* described him as '... a delightful host and guest, having a rich fund of humour'. A warm appreciation was included by Sir Leon Radzinowicz in the preface he contributed to *Camps on Crime*, published in 1973. He wrote that his friend was '... constantly opening out broader vistas, more human perspectives ...', and he summarised Camps's philosophy of investigation, 'as hard work, attention to detail and emotional detachment.'

Chapter Five

THE TEACHER

Keith Simpson

KEITH SIMPSON WAS FASCINATED BY DEATH, which is perhaps not surprising for a forensic pathologist. But his interest was more introspective than simply a doctor's pronouncement about the extinction of life. He considered the moral issues raised by medical procedures which might prolong life to a point where the body no longer has the capacity to survive by itself. Treatment of terminal cancer and determination of brain death in organ donors pose weighty questions for medical practitioners.

These were not normally matters for the forensic pathologist whose subjects were beyond such considerations, but the issues involved concerned Keith Simpson. In an essay entitled, *Moment of Death*, published in 1967, he asked whether there were historic examples of people declared dead and subsequently found to be alive. 'Is it possible?' he asked, and answered, 'undeniably, yes,' quoting the case of a woman who supposedly committed suicide but was found to be breathing when her body arrived at the mortuary. He committed these and related thoughts to print a year after his wife, Mary, to whom he had been married for twenty-three years, died of multiple sclerosis. Death and the bearing of it must have been very much in his mind.

He could also turn these questions on their head by adding a dash of black humour to accounts of his work when he was invited to talk to clubs and societies where he was a popular speaker. One of his favourite stories concerned a post-mortem he carried out on an elderly man who, in life, suffered from curvature of the spine, resulting in a pronounced stoop. In order to make the corpse lay flat in its coffin, Simpson straightened the backbone using a length of metal tubing. All went well until the coffin was consigned to the flames of the crematorium oven. Subjected to intense heat, the metal tube in the corpse buckled, with the result that the dead man rose up through the burning coffin. Simpson liked to tease his audience by asking them how they thought the crematorium staff might have reacted.

Keith Simpson was born in Brighton where his father practised as a GP. In his autobiography, he wrote, 'I became a doctor because my father was one.' With his future direction clearly identified, he prospered at school and, at the age of seventeen, enrolled at Guy's Medical School in 1924. He admired his teachers and the idea of passing on and sharing learning and knowledge to others would be a strong thread in his subsequent career. After qualifying in medicine, he elected to pursue pathology and was appointed as Demonstrator in Pathology at Guy's in 1932. In the same year, he married Mary Buchanan who was a hospital nurse.

Two years later, he was appointed Supervisor of medico-legal post-mortems and, subsequently, became an adviser to the Surrey Police. The world of forensic pathology at that time, at least in England, was dominated by the presence of Sir Bernard Spilsbury. Good-looking and firm of jaw, he captured the headlines but kept his distance from his fellow professionals and the natural camaraderie which normally exists in such groups. Simpson would later refer to Spilsbury, rather uncharitably, as, 'unloved and unmourned'. A trio of pathologists, Donald Teare, Francis Camps and Simpson, served the needs of London in the medical investigation of suspicious deaths. They were affectionately known to the police as 'The Three Musketeers', and, even during the early war years and the London Blitz, they met regularly for lunch in a Soho restaurant to compare notes and cases.

In 1941, Simpson engaged a secretary, Molly Lefebure, who worked for him throughout the Second World War and proved a valuable assistant. She came from a journalistic background and, being fairly worldly-wise, made the transition from newspaper office to mortuary reporting with ease. Unlike Spilsbury, who would not employ a secretary and made handwritten notes of his cases, Simpson relied on his secretary, who acted very much like a modern personal assistant. His first big case – his Crippen moment – came in 1942. On 17 July, a workman clearing debris from a blitzed church in south London unearthed a skeleton which he imagined was the remains of a victim of the German bombing. He put the body parts to one side while he finished his task and, in due course, reported the discovery to his foreman.

The following day, Dr Simpson was asked by the police to examine the remains which had been taken to the mortuary at Southwark. The presence of a womb in the abdominal cavity determined the sex of the body. His first assessment of the age of the fire-blackened remains was between a year and eighteen months. He viewed the circumstances of the discovery as puzzling. The body had been found buried beneath a stone slab in a cellar floor; not at all like a bomb-damage casualty. And the church had been blitzed in August 1940 which did not correspond with the preliminary assessment of the length of time the body had been dead. Simpson was given permission by the coroner to take the remains back to his laboratory at Guy's where he could carry out a more thorough examination.

He established that parts of the arms and legs were missing and, subsequently, returned to the bombed-out church to see if any further bones might come to light. Despite the removal of nearly three tons of earth, no human bone fragments were found, but the pathologist's attention was caught by the presence of yellowish deposits in the cellar and a wooden box. Analysis showed that the deposit was slaked lime. Suspicions formed that the body might have been brought in the box to the cellar where it was buried in lime. Murder was very much on the cards and this line of thought was strengthened by the pathologist's examination of what remained of the limbs on the skeleton. Both legs had been cut off at the knee and the arms severed at the elbow; clear indications of dismemberment.

It was the teeth remaining in the upper jaw which provided evidence of identity. Simpson had already alerted the police to this possibility when officers trawled through lists of missing persons and found the name of Rachel Dobkin. She was the wife of a fire watcher and had been reported missing by her sister. The description she provided broadly matched what was known about the dead woman and, most importantly, she knew the name of Rachel Dobkin's dentist. It was a short step to invite the dentist to view the teeth in the jaw. He recognised his work immediately and amid much excitement, declared 'That's my patient . . . That's Mrs Dobkin.'

Armed with a family photograph of Rachel Dobkin, Dr Simpson set about superimposing the facial image onto a photograph of the skull. This was a technique employed with considerable success a few years earlier by John Glaister and Professor Brash in the Ruxton case. Working with the photographic technician at Guy's, Simpson prepared a positive image of Dobkin's portrait and a negative image of the skull on transparent X-ray film and placed one over the other. 'The portrait fitted the skull like a mask,' he wrote later. The remains found in the bomb-damaged church were those of Rachel Dobkin. This was a moment of triumph for the young pathologist in what his secretary, Molly Lefebure, described as a 'case of a lifetime'. To add a further shine to his work, Simpson had retrieved the remains of a larynx preserved in the lime at the scene of burial. He found that the thyroid cartilage was broken and surrounded by a blood clot. This was firm evidence that Rachel Dobkin had been strangled.

The conclusion of the case was left to the police who located Harry Dobkin and invited him to answer a few questions about his wife's disappearance. As a result, he was charged with murder and sent for trial at the Old Bailey. The jury took twenty minutes to find him guilty and he was subsequently executed at Wandsworth Prison. In the final act of what had been a remarkable case, Simpson carried out the post-mortem on the executed man's corpse. Molly Lefebure recorded that Dobkin, '. . . looked very peaceful. His debts were settled at last', she said. Simpson concluded, a touch ruefully, that if there had not been a war on, his case might have achieved headlines to match those that Spilsbury had achieved with Crippen.

Investigation of another concealed burial came to Dr Simpson's attention just a few months after the first. In October 1942, soldiers on manoeuvres at Hankley Common near Godalming in Surrey came across a body buried in a shallow grave. All that was visible was a hand rising up through the earth as if beckoning attention. Simpson was called to the scene and the outstretched body of a young woman was uncovered. The maggot-strewn corpse was clothed and lying face down. The massive injury to the back of the skull was all too apparent. The remains were taken to Guy's Hospital for further examination.

The corpse was that of a woman aged around nineteen to twenty who was identified by her clothing. She was known to the police on account of the fact that she lived rough on Hankley Common in a wigwam made from tree branches and foliage. This shelter had been made for her by a Canadian soldier based at Witley Camp who was her boyfriend. August Sangret, aged thirty, was a French-Canadian of native North American stock. Simpson determined that the woman's skull had been smashed with a violent blow, probably from a tree branch used as a bludgeon. The presence of adipocere on the body led him to estimate that Pearl Wolfe had been dead for between five and seven weeks. The broken skull, which had fractured into thirty-eight pieces, was re-assembled in the laboratory with help from Dr Eric Gardner, whom Simpson liked to call a 'GP pathologist'. They found two stab wounds which had penetrated the bone. There were also defensive wounds on one of the arms. A characteristic of the stab wounds was that they seemed to have been inflicted with a knife having a distinctive hooked blade.

A detailed search of the area where the body was found turned up a tree branch with hair impacted on one end. The microscopic characteristics of the hair matched the head hair of the dead woman and the thickness of the branch corresponded with the skull injury. Simpson had no doubt that this was the murder weapon. His reconstruction of the crime was that Pearl Wolfe had been stabbed but managed to escape her attacker until he caught up and smashed her skull with the tree branch. He then dragged the body to the place where it was buried, causing injuries to her legs. The question was, where was the knife?

August Sangret was questioned and made a long, rambling statement. He admitted his liaison with Pearl Wolfe and it emerged later that he had reported to his regimental Provost Sergeant that she had failed to turn up for a pre-arranged meeting. The Sergeant told Sangret that this was a private matter and no business of his, to which Sangret responded, tellingly, by saying, 'If she's found and anything has happened to her, I don't want to be mixed up in it.' The soldier's uniform and blankets were examined by detectives and proved to have been recently washed but there was no knife among his personal effects. By chance, a soldier picking blackberries on Hankley Common found a knife stuck in a tree close to a shack used by Sangret. The soldier handed the knife in to the regimental provosts who described it as British Army issue with a black handle and hooked blade. As the knife was found near Sangret's shack, he was given the chance to claim ownership and promptly accepted.

The next time the knife appeared, it was by another chance discovery, this time as the result of unblocking a drain. A soldier clearing a drain at Witley Camp retrieved a black-handled knife with a hooked blade. When Simpson examined it, he found no incriminating fingerprints but determined that the blade fitted perfectly into the holes that Pearl Wolfe's attacker had stabbed into her skull. Sangret was charged with murder and sent for trial at Kingston Assizes. The pathologist attended to give expert evidence, equipped with the murder victim's skull and the hook-bladed knife. He demonstrated to the court how precisely the knife fitted into the skull injuries and, when the jury retired, they took both articles with them. After two hours' deliberation, they found August Sangret guilty but with a recommendation to mercy. The recommendation was not acted upon and the convicted soldier was executed at Wandsworth Prison. Once again, Simpson had the last word when he carried out the post-mortem following Sangret's execution.

Many years later, in 1978, when the *Sunday Telegraph* serialised Keith Simpson's autobiography, *Forty Years of Murder*, the pathologist posed for a photograph to be shown on the cover of the magazine. It was a reprise of his appearance in court over thirty years earlier; looking slightly menacing, he held the murder knife in one hand and the victim's skull in the other. It was publicity of a type that Spilsbury could not have imagined.

'The Three Musketeers' continued to deal with the dead in London and the Home Counties. They were not all headline cases with suspicion attached, but simply corpses requiring confirmation of cause of death. As Molly Lefebure recorded in her memoir, *Evidence for the Crown*, published in 1954, her boss was carrying out between ten and twenty-eight post-mortems a day. Where there was no need of extended investigation, Keith Simpson would often complete seven or eight examinations in a morning. Even with the steady flow of bodies, lecturing duties at Guy's, air-raid warnings and raising a family, he still found time to write. The first edition of his textbook, *Forensic Medicine*, was published in 1947.

War, or no war, it seemed that people were still driven to commit murder on the domestic front for the time-honoured motives of elimination, revenge and jealousy. Following his success in establishing the victim's identity in the Dobkin case, Keith Simpson was soon confronted with another identification puzzle. Workers changing shifts at the Vauxhall car factory in Luton on 19 November 1943 followed a familiar route, walking along the towpath which ran beside the River Lea, on their way to the factory gates. Some of them noticed a bundle lying in the reeds of the shallow, murky river but thought no more of it. Later that day, two Luton Corporation employees also observed the bundle when they made routine checks on the water levels. They waded out into the river and pulled the bundle open sufficiently to see what was inside. They recoiled in horror when their curiosity was rewarded by the sight of a pale, bloodied face of a woman.

When the police arrived on the scene, the bundle was pulled up onto the river bank for closer inspection. The naked body of a woman was revealed and her battered face showed that she had been the victim of a violent attack. The police surgeon looked at the facial injuries and mistakenly determined that the woman had been shot. He arranged for the body to be taken to the mortuary at Luton and Dunstable Hospital pending the arrival of the Home Office pathologist, Dr Keith Simpson. He carried out a post-mortem examination on the corpse which he judged to be a female aged between thirty and thirty-five. She was about five feet, three inches tall and her body had been doubled up and enclosed in four sacks. Her ankles had been tied together and the knees bound to her chest. Bruises on her back suggested she might have been pinned down in at attempt at strangulation, but that was not the cause of death. There were massive injuries to the face, including a split cheek, fractured jaw, a wound across one eye and another injury that had practically severed an ear. There were bruises on the elbows and hands, suggesting a struggle had taken place. The pathologist found vital reaction in bruises on the legs which he thought might indicate she was concussed following the heavy blows to the face but, not at that point, dead. The woman was five and a half months pregnant.

Simpson estimated that death had occurred thirty to forty minutes after the head injuries had been inflicted. The body had not been in the water longer than twenty-four hours. There was no jewellery on it and no distinguishing marks, although a denture appeared to be missing. At this stage, the victim was simply a Jane Doe. The police investigation was led by Chief Inspector William Chapman who organised a painstaking search of the scene. The river bed was dragged and the banks searched. Missing Persons Lists were consulted, house-to-house enquiries made and workers at the Vauxhall factory interviewed to determine if any of them had noticed signs of suspicious activity anywhere on the riverside. The dead woman's identity proved elusive. There was no match for her finger-prints in criminal records so it was decided to circulate photographs of her face. This was not a decision arrived at easily because her features had been battered almost beyond recognition. Nevertheless, police photographers came up with a passable side portrait view which was published in the local newspaper in the hope that someone would recognise her and come forward with a name. The photograph was also shown at local cinemas and, as a result of this publicity, several people came forward and were invited to view the body although no positive identification resulted.

Chief Inspector Chapman decided to widen his search activities to include trawling through street refuse bins and council rubbish tips. This unappealing task finally rewarded searchers with a possible clue in the form of a fragment of clothing bearing a dry-cleaning label. The remnant of a black coat was traced to a dry-cleaning shop whose records showed that the garment belonged to Mrs Caroline Manton who lived in Regent Street, Luton.

DCI Chapman called at the house and his knock on the door was answered by a young girl. He asked if her mother was at home, to which the child's response was that her mother had gone away. The detective's instinct told him he was on the right track and, not least, because the girl bore a startling likeness to the dead woman's photograph. He had also gleaned information about the girl's grandmother whom he arranged to visit. Elderly Mrs Bavister provided him with evidence which would prove to be significant. The late Mrs Manton's mother mentioned that she had received four letters from her daughter during the three months that she had been missing. The astute detective noticed various spelling mistakes in the writing and his keen eye was drawn to a missing letter 'p' in the word, 'Hamstead'. His next port of call was to revisit the Manton family home where he intended to question Bertie Manton, the dead woman's husband. He worked in the National Fire Service and was on duty in Luton when the detective called. Chapman located him at his fire station and learned that he was trapped in an unhappy marriage to Caroline, also known as Rene, and that they had quarrelled, allegedly over her extra-marital affairs. Manton said they parted company on 25 November when Rene left home and went to stay with relatives.

He professed not to recognise her from the police photograph he was shown, but identified as hers the handwriting in the letters received by her mother. The detective then asked Manton to write out a sentence which he indicated in one of the letters supposedly sent by his wife to her mother. This he did and, with Chapman looking over his shoulder, he spelled the word 'Hampstead' without its letter 'p'. The final question the policeman asked Manton was the name of Rene's dentist, which was readily supplied. When, in due course, the dentist was shown the photograph of Rene Manton, he instantly recognised her as a patient for whom he had fitted a denture in May 1943. Identification was placed beyond doubt when the patient's dental records were matched to the dentition in the jaw of the dead woman.

When Manton was arrested and charged with murder, he promptly confessed. He apologised for lying when previously questioned and admitted killing his wife, although he explained that he had not intended to do so: 'I lost my temper,' he said. He told detectives that there had been a marital argument during lunch on 18 November when Rene threw a cup of hot tea into his face. At this point, he lost his temper and, picking up a heavy wooden stool, smashed it several times against her head. When his anger abated, he realised he had killed her and decided to hide the body and tidy up before his children returned from school. He stripped her clothes off, removed her jewellery and took the body down to the cellar as a temporary hiding place. To earn a little extra money to supplement his fireman's wages, Manton ran a small greengrocery business from home for which he kept a supply of potato sacks. He now used four of these to conceal the body after tying it up at the knees and ankles. Manton then cleaned up the bloodstains and when his children returned home asking for their mother, he told them she had gone to stay with grandma.

After their evening meal, his eldest daughter went to visit a friend and Manton gave the other three children money to go to the cinema. While they were absent from the house and as darkness fell, he brought the body up from the cellar, balanced the sacked-up bundle over the handlebars of his bicycle and pushed it down the road towards the River Lea where he rolled it down the bank and into the water. In his statement, he said, 'I then rode home and got the children's supper ready. They never suspected anything.' When detectives searched the house they found bloodstains in the living room which tested as Group O, the same as Mrs Manton. The noted fingerprint sleuth, Superintendent Fred Cherrill, did a search for prints and found one on an empty pickle jar. It matched Mrs Manton's left thumb and, as Keith Simpson put it very succinctly, 'That clinched the identification.'

While Bertie Manton's cleaning-up operations had been well organised, they were not quite foolproof. He had been careful to dispose of the murder weapon, the wooden footstool, which he had broken up for firewood, but he had left sufficient blood traces in the house to enable crime technicians to match blood groups. Crucially, he did not burn his wife's coat when he was clearing her clothes but cut it into pieces for disposal with the household refuse. When part of it turned up during the police fingertip searches and it was identified as belonging to Caroline Manton, his game was up.

Manton was sent for trial at Bedford Assizes in May 1944. His defence was manslaughter, argued along the lines that he was a mild-mannered man provoked by his wife who had strayed into the company of other men and taken to drink. His wife's death was not premeditated and the extensive cover up he engaged in was for the benefit of his children. Keith Simpson's evidence was telling, for he said he had found clear indications of an attempt to strangle Mrs Manton. The defendant's response to this was that he remembered, 'taking hold of her throat and pushing her against the wall. I may have grabbed her twice, but that was in my temper.' This was an admission he had not previously made and it went a long way to ensure his conviction. Simpson described the outcome as, 'a strangling and bashing murder'. He also reserved some scathing remarks, expressed privately, about the police surgeon who had first examined Mrs Manton's body and could not distinguish blunt force trauma from gunshot wounds. The jury found Manton guilty and Mr Justice Singleton sentenced him to hang.

Despite the brutal nature of his crime, Manton had garnered considerable public sympathy and a petition for mercy collected 30,000 signatures. One of his young sons campaigned on his father's behalf and sentence was commuted to life imprisonment on appeal. Manton became ill in prison and died at Parkhurst in November 1947. The investigation of this case had, once again, shown the invaluable nature of dental evidence in establishing identity. This was an area of forensic work in which Simpson was a pioneering influence. Credit was also due in the 'Luton Sack Murder' to the meticulous attention to detail demonstrated by Detective Inspector Chapman.

Keith Simpson had the dubious privilege of being involved in three of the most infamous post-war murder cases. In the early 1950s, one of the tour guides at St Paul's Cathedral who conducted visitors around the 'Whispering Gallery' in the dome, regaled them with stories of London criminals. ''Eath, 'Aigh and Christie,' he would say, 'I knew 'em all!' It was an idle boast but it captivated his audiences. He was, of course, referring to the notorious trio, Neville Heath, John Haigh and John Christie and, although he did not brag about it, Keith Simpson did know them all in his own inimitable way.

When the chambermaid failed to obtain a response from the occupants of Room Number 4 at the Pembridge Court Hotel in Notting Hill Gate on 21 June 1946, she used a pass key to gain entry. The double room was booked in the names of Lieutenant Colonel and Mrs N.G.C. Heath. The maid saw a woman lying in bed on her back, with the sheet drawn up to her neck. She sensed that something was wrong and sent for the manager. When the sheet was pulled back, they found themselves looking at a mutilated body. The dead woman was the sole occupant of the room; there was no sign of 'Lt-Col Heath'. The police were called and Superintendent Fred Cherrill lost no time in telephoning Dr Simpson. The pathologist examined the body and found extensive bite marks on the woman's breasts and her ankles were bound together, effectively hiding a savage injury to her vagina. It was clear from bruises on her wrists that she had been tied hand and foot. Turning the body over, he found that she had been savagely whipped across her back, with seventeen separate lash marks evident. Simpson determined that the injuries had been inflicted while the victim was still alive. Cause of death was suffocation, possibly due to being gagged.

The dead woman was identified as thirty-two-year-old Margery Gardner and hotel staff were well acquainted with her companion, 'Lt-Col Heath', who had stayed at the hotel before. Conscious of the need to find the sexual sadist who had committed this savage murder, the police quickly identified their target as Neville Heath and a description of him was issued to the press. Simpson had made a close examination of the whip marks on Gardner's body and noted the diamond-shaped pattern made on the skin. 'If you find that whip,' he told Superintendent Cherrill, 'you've found your man'.

Neville Heath, meanwhile, had booked into the Tollard Royal Hotel at Bournemouth, using the name Group Captain Rupert Brooke. On 5 July, Doreen Marshall who had been staying at the Norfolk Hotel in the town was reported missing. When last seen, she left the hotel in a taxi heading for the Tollard Royal for dinner. Enquiries established that she might have dined with Group Captain Rupert Brooke. When asked about his companion, the Group Captain glossed over the matter by saying he had known the lady for years. Then, in an extraordinary move, he contacted the local police asking to see a photograph of the missing woman. He called in at the police station and identified a photograph of Doreen Marshall, confirming that she had dined with him a few nights before. At this point, 'Group Captain Brooke' was identified as Neville Heath. When he was searched, a cloakroom ticket issued at Bournemouth West railway station was found in his coat pocket. The ticket was for a suitcase which was quickly redeemed and opened. In it were a bloodstained scarf and a distinctive leather whip which bore out Dr Simpson's earlier advice to police.

On 8 July, the body of Doreen Marshall was found in bushes at Branscombe Dene Chine about a mile from central Bournemouth. She had been brutally attacked and mutilated, with her sexual organs particularly targeted. She had died from a cut throat and the worst injuries had been inflicted after death. A local pathologist carried out the post-mortem but Simpson gained possession of the contents of Heath's suitcase. Speaking of the injuries inflicted on Margery Gardner, the pathologist wrote later, 'If ever I saw a murderer's signature on his handiwork it was the imprint . . . of the riding whip with the diamond patterned weave.' Justice caught up with Neville Heath and a defence plea of insanity did not save him from the scaffold. He was hanged on 16 October 1946.

By this time, Molly Lefebure had left Simpson's employment in order to get married. He replaced her with Jean Scott-Dunn whom he would eventually marry. Sadness had earlier intruded in his life with the illness which struck down his first wife, Mary Buchanan, who died of multiple sclerosis in 1955. Personal life apart, the bodies kept on coming and, in 1949, came the Haigh murder case which was another of those 'once in a lifetime' episodes. Like Neville Heath, John George Haigh, a self-styled engineer, was regarded as a gentleman charmer. He lived in a Kensington hotel where the residents, mostly rich elderly widows, doted on him. On 18 February, he invited wealthy sixty-nine-year-old Olive Durand-Deacon to visit his factory in Crawley, Sussex, where he manufactured artificial fingernails for the cosmetics trade. In reality, his factory was nothing more than a storeroom and yard.

When Mrs Durand-Deacon failed to return from her trip to Sussex, alarm bells started to sound about her safety. The mention of Haigh's name as a person with whom she had consorted, led detectives to check the criminal records at Scotland Yard. Officers discovered that Haigh had 'previous' with convictions for fraud and shady dealing, although there were no suggestions of violent crimes. Sussex Police decided to search Haigh's factory premises and they made some interesting discoveries. They found a .38 revolver and ammunition, large quantities of sulphuric acid and an assortment of protective clothing. Also found was a dry-cleaner's receipt dated 19 February, the day Mrs Durand-Deacon disappeared, for a Persian lamb coat. This created suspicion, for it was known that the missing woman was wearing such a coat when last seen. When her jewellery was reported as having been sold, detectives decided it was time to invite Mr Haigh to answer some questions.

In an extraordinary interview, Haigh volunteered the information that Mrs Durand-Deacon 'no longer exists. She has disappeared completely and no trace of her can ever be found again'. It was a bold statement but he had reckoned without the pertinacity of Keith Simpson. Haigh admitted destroying Mrs Durand-Deacon with acid and challenged the police with the statement, 'How can you prove murder if there is no body?' This was the second pronouncement he had made that would come back to haunt him. Haigh completed his admissions in a lengthy statement in which he confessed to the murders of five other people whose bodies he had destroyed with acid. He claimed in each case to have drunk a glass of his victim's blood, thereby allowing newspaper editors to include the word 'vampire' in their headlines.

At this point, Keith Simpson entered the investigation. With the knowledge that the murder victims had been disposed of in vats of sulphuric acid, he turned over in his mind what might be left after such a corrosive assault. On arrival at Haigh's factory, his attention was drawn to an area in the yard where one of the acid vats had been emptied onto the ground. Among the debris on the surface, his eagle eye spotted a small faceted stone. He nonchalantly remarked to the police Inspector on hand, 'I think that's a gallstone.' Part of his mental preparation for the visit to Crawley was the knowledge that a person of Mrs Durand-Deacon's age might well have gallstones lodged in her body which, covered with fatty tissue, would survive the destructive potential of sulphuric acid.

Detailed examination of a mass of greasy sludge resulted in the discovery of several small pieces of bone of human origin and, most significantly, he found a set of acrylic dentures. These too had survived the acid test and the teeth were unquestionably identified as Mrs Durand-Deacon's by her dentist who had fitted them for her in September 1947. Simpson had without doubt discovered what little remained of the murder victim. Haigh was committed for trial at Lewes Assizes where much of the evidence concerned his state of mind. He pleaded not guilty by reason of insanity. Dr Henry Yellowlees, a distinguished psychiatrist, had diagnosed Haigh as paranoic, but said he was fully responsible under the law. In essence, he was not insane, which was the conclusion the jury arrived at.

After deliberating for just eighteen minutes, they found Haigh sane and guilty. He was executed at Wandsworth on 10 August 1949.

Writing about the case in his book, *The Mind of the Murderer*, published in 1957, Dr W.L. Neustatter, a leading forensic psychiatrist, referred to Haigh as a malingerer and 'simulator of insanity', suggesting he was either insane, psychopathic or simply plausible, clever and wicked. Whatever his state of mind, he clearly established a place for himself in the annals of crime as the 'Acid Bath Murderer'. But for the astute observations of Keith Simpson, Haigh's crimes might have remained unsolved. There were also some interesting parallels with the Luton Sack Murder, notably the important part played by dental evidence, and the telltale significance of a dry-cleaning ticket.

By the time that the Haigh case came to trial, Spilsbury had departed the stage. The commanding influence which he had exerted for over thirty years died with him, for above all else, he was a loner. His death opened the way for a new approach to forensic medicine and 'The Three Musketeers' began to think about a collective approach to forensic work. To that end, in 1950 they established the Association in Forensic Medicine and Sir Sydney Smith accepted the invitation to become its first President. There was also a new emphasis on teaching, and professorships in forensic medicine were set up by London University. Keith Simpson became the first Professor of Forensic Medicine at Guy's in 1962 and Francis Camps occupied the chair at the London Hospital Medical College in 1963. This show of unity was to prove short-lived, though, as Camps had a tendency to break ranks by appearing in court giving expert testimony in opposition to his colleagues.

The only occasion 'The Three Musketeers' appeared together on the same case was during the investigation of the murders at 10 Rillington Place. The exhumation of Timothy Evan's wife and daughter in 1953 brought the trio together under the roof of Kensington Mortuary. Donald Teare had conducted the original post-mortem examinations eight years previously but the re-examination of the exhumed bodies was undertaken by Camps, acting on instructions from the Attorney-General, while Simpson represented the interests of John Christie, who was the self-confessed murderer. Christie's trial was the third post-war headline-grabbing criminal case after Heath and Haigh. An account of the proceedings is given in Chapter Four, suffice it to say here that the meeting of the country's three most eminent pathologists was marred by an unseemly squabble about taking tissues for laboratory tests from the exhumed corpses. Camps resented Simpson's insistence on testing Geraldine Evans's body for traces of carbon monoxide poisoning. Relations between Simpson and Camps had reached a turning point and their dealings became increasingly fractured after this incident. In 1958, Camps broke with the wartime triumvirate and set up his British Academy of Forensic Sciences.

A case which quickly acquired newspaper headlines was 'The Chalkpit Murder' and it inspired what Keith Simpson described as 'one of the mysteries of medico-legal history'. Late in the afternoon of 30 November 1946, a man walking past an old chalk pit near Woldingham in Surrey saw a body lying in a shallow, open trench which was a relic of wartime military manoeuvres. He called the police who were soon at the scene, followed by Dr Eric Gardner, consultant patholo-gist at Weybridge Hospital, who examined the corpse with the aid of a torch. He noted a noose around the neck and ascertained that the man had been dead for forty-eight hours. The following morning, with the benefit of daylight, Dr Gardner, in the company of Keith Simpson, who was acting as a consultant to the Surrey Police, took a more detailed look at the body. Simpson's immediate reaction was that it looked like an '. . . open-and-shut case of murder. The dead man's face was plum-coloured and he had a noose around his neck.' He observed that, despite recent heavy rain which had turned the ground into mud, the dead man's shoes were completely clean. The clothes on the upper part of the body were bunched up, suggesting that the body might have been dragged by the feet and placed in the trench. There were indications that an attempt had been made to bury the body with loose soil and a pickaxe was found nearby.

The corpse was taken to Oxted Mortuary where Dr Gardner carried out a post-mortem examination under the observant scrutiny of Keith Simpson. Evidence of asphyxia was apparent in small petechial haemorrhages in the eyes and face. Internal examination showed congestion in all the organs. Particular attention was focussed on the neck which was encircled by a marked groove. Two pieces of rope and a piece of green cloth were fixed loosely around the neck in a half-hitch with several feet of rope to spare. As Simpson recorded later, if the rope mark had been horizontal, it would have suggested strangulation with a ligature. But the mark was most evident low on the right side and high on the left part of the neck where it came up under the ear. His conclusion was that this was a death by hanging. The experienced pathologist knew that hanging rarely meant murder; it was invariably indicative of suicide. There were no indications of a struggle having taken place which led the two doctors to agree, at that stage, the likely scenario was of a man who had hanged himself.

The circumstances in which self-suspension might have occurred raised a differ-ent set of questions. Post-mortem lividity and rigor mortis indicated that the body had entered the trench where it was found soon after death. But how did it get there? One possibility was that the man had hanged himself from a nearby tree and fallen, or slid down, into the trench where he died. The police looked in vain for marks on any trees close by which might have served as a suspension point and, of course, there was also the matter of the clean shoes to be taken into account.

The dead man had been identified as thirty-five-year-old John McBain Mudie, a hotel barman from Reigate, who had been missing for two days. A trawl through Mudie's personal effects produced a letter requesting the return of some cheques to a property company. This opened up a complex trail of investigation, starting with the Chairman of Connaught Properties Limited, Thomas John Ley. He was interviewed by a detective on 8 December at his house in Kensington. Sixty-six-year-old Ley had emigrated to Australia as a boy where he eventually entered politics and became Minister of Justice in 1922. He returned to England in 1929 and he pursued various business interests. Ley explained the background to the letter sent to John Mudie and the detective went away satisfied that his enquiries had been adequately answered.

Following press reports that a body had been found near Woldingham, two men informed the police that, on their way home from work on 30 November, they had seen a man standing by the chalk pit. When he spotted them, he ran off towards a parked car and drove away. They remembered that '101' was part of the car's registration number. The next episode in this rapidly developing investigation occurred when an ex-boxer, John William Buckingham, came forward with information. He told the police that he operated a car for hire and had been asked to get in contact with a Mr Ley who was prepared to pay a large sum to a driver who could keep his mouth shut. Buckingham did as he was asked and Ley explained that in his role as a solicitor he was protecting two women who were being blackmailed by a man named Jack Mudie. He wanted Mudie brought to his London home so that he could deal with the matter. Also present during this discussion was Lawrence John Smith who acted as Ley's odd-job man.

The story unfolded that, on 28 November, Mudie was delivered to Ley's home where a blanket was put over his head and Smith tied him up. Buckingham, his part in this incident completed, departed with an envelope containing £200. He saw Smith a few days later who told him that Mr Ley was very satisfied with the way things had gone and that Mudie had been paid to leave the country. Scotland Yard officers interviewed Smith on 17 December when he made a voluntary statement admitting the part he had played in helping Buckingham to kidnap Mudie. When he was questioned, Ley simply denied everything.

By now, the police had located the car, registration number FGP 101, which Smith had hired and he was identified by the two men who had seen someone standing near the chalk pit. On 28 December, Ley, Buckingham and Smith were arrested and charged with murder. The conundrum of how precisely Mudie had met his death deepened at this point, because Keith Simpson felt there was a drift towards defining the medical evidence in a way that supported a murder charge. In taking this view, he was at odds with his friend and colleague, Eric Gardner, who, in due course, would give expert testimony for the prosecution. Simpson feared that a miscarriage of justice might result if Gardner's evidence went unchallenged. The scene was thus set for confrontation and a further development ensued when Buckingham agreed to give evidence for the prosecution against the other two defendants.

Dr Gardner's evidence given at the magistrates' court was confined to the serious injuries which he believed Mudie had sustained in a struggle, chief of which he believed was a blow to the head. In his later recollections, Keith Simpson mentioned that he was not called upon to present his findings at the committal proceedings, although defence lawyers were fully aware of his views. He added, drily, that after they had read his post-mortem report, 'they audaciously invited me to change sides'. Ley and Smith, who pleaded not guilty to the charges, were committed for trial at the Old Bailey. Simpson did not normally offer his services to the defence in criminal trials but, in this instance, he was prepared to make an exception. As it turned out, he found himself on the same side as Francis Camps who had already been enrolled by the defence team.

The trial opened on 19 March 1947 before Lord Chief Justice Goddard. In his account of the trial, the editor of the *Medico-Legal Journal* mentioned the appearance of the two men in the dock; 'Ley, prosperous and well-dressed, portly, square headed with a bulbous nose, looked almost as if he were presiding at a company meeting.' By contrast, Smith was, 'obviously a working man' and 'ill at ease'. While Camps did little more than describe the post-mortem effects of asphyxia, Simpson was given a hard time under cross-examination and not least by Lord Goddard. He was insistent that the rope around the victim's neck which caused the asphyxia was drawn and lifted. In answer to prosecuting counsel, he said, that lifting 'was the significant thing . . .'.

'Why?' asked counsel.

'Because,' replied Simpson, '. . . it wouldn't necessarily cause death; it was the lifting that did it.'

Badgered by Lord Goddard, Simpson refused to give ground on his interpretation of the facts as he understood them. He reiterated that the dead man had been found with a rope around his neck which had been pulled tight and lifted, killing him in the process. He refused to speculate on the circumstances beyond agreeing that the victim had been suspended in some way, adding, 'we have no evidence.' Lord Goddard commented acidly, 'Well, at any rate, we have got as far as that.' In his biography of Lord Goddard, published in 1977, Fenton Bresler remarked on Simpson's 'remarkable stand for scientific integrity, committing himself solely within the confines of his own specific knowledge.'

Dr Gardner was examined in considerable detail about the pathological appearances of asphyxia, and the textbook opinions of both Spilsbury and Glaister were cited. His position, in essence, was that Mudie was strangled by a rope placed around his neck which caused slow strangulation. He contended that the mark left by the rope indicated some form of suspension not involving a drop. His view was that the rope might have been pulled up when the unconscious victim was in a sagging position. His precise words were, 'I mean, if the loop of that rope were over the knob of the chair, you have got the ideal position.' In his summing up, Lord Goddard told the jury that he did not propose to discuss which of the two doctors' opinions was correct, stating that the victim was killed by being strangled by a rope with some upward movement of suspension. The Lord Chief Justice drew a picture of how a man might be sitting in a chair with someone behind him pulling on a rope around his neck and strangling him. That, he said, 'would be a degree of suspension'. He sent the jury out to consider their verdict at 4.35 p.m. and they were back in the courtroom within an hour to deliver guilty verdicts on both Ley and Smith. The pair were sentenced to death after Ley complained about what he termed the judge's biased summing up. It might be said that the former Minister of Justice had his day in court.

On 5 May 1947, Thomas Ley was reprieved by the Home Secretary after he was declared insane and committed to Broadmoor, while Smith's sentence was reduced to life imprisonment. Ley died a couple of months later from a stroke and Eric Gardner, who had been suffering from tuberculosis, died in 1951. Keith Simpson had been critical of his friend who he believed had, 'stuck out his neck unnecessarily' and thereby highlighted the problem of trying too assiduously to help the police. It seemed that the desire to seek truth and justice strained their relationship but Simpson said they remained close friends.

Breaking the sequence of the big post-war murder cases was an episode which enabled Simpson, justifiably, to claim a forensic first. The murder of Margaret Gorringe in Kent in 1948 provided the pathologist with evidence of bite marks on her body which led him to believe he could identify her attacker. The bites were made by an individual whose teeth were unevenly spaced and curiously angled. Suspicion fell on the dead woman's husband and it was known that the couple had quarrelled. As there was no dentist available, Simpson himself took a cast of the suspect's teeth and showed that the impressions matched the bite marks on the body in every detail. In due course, Gorringe was convicted of murdering his wife and, in his quiet way, the pathologist had chalked up the first identification of a murderer in Britain by teeth marks left on the victim's body.

The pathologist commented on the lack of interest in forensic dentistry in Britain, although studies were well advanced in Sweden and the USA. In particular, Dr Gösta Gustafson, working at Lund University, developed techniques for estimating the age of an individual from the teeth. His work on *Forensic Odontology*, published in 1966, was a landmark textbook. Simpson's own achievements had not gone unnoticed, though, for colleagues in Scotland sought his help with a case in 1967 when a teenage girl was reported missing from her home in the village of Biggar in Scotland. When fifteen-year-old Linda Peacock had not returned home by 11 p.m. on Sunday 6 August, local police mounted a search.

Early the following morning, Linda's body was found lying in the graveyard of St Mary's Church. She appeared to have been strangled during a sexually motivated attack in which she suffered head wounds. Of particular significance was a bite mark on her right breast. A police task force under the command of Chief Superintendent William Muncie, made house-to-house and other enquiries. These were passed through what he called 'the sieve', including initial checks at a nearby boys' school. Meanwhile, a photograph of the bite mark on the girl's breast was sent to the Department of Forensic Dentistry at the Police Training School in Liverpool. The assessment made was that the marks could be used both to eliminate suspects and also to identify the attacker.

Dr Warren Harvey, consultant at Glasgow Dental Hospital, who was on holiday in Ireland, was sent a copy of the photograph and he responded by confirming the importance of bite mark evidence to the enquiry. A breakthrough came when one of the boys at the school in Biggar admitted giving false information to the police about the absence of one of his fellow pupils, seventeen-year-old Gordon Hay. It now appeared that Hay had returned to his dormitory in an excited state late on Sunday evening and persuaded his friends to tell detectives that they were all in bed, including himself, by 10 p.m.

By this time, Hay had been transferred to another school but officers interviewed him and brought him back to Biggar. He denied knowing Linda Peacock and insisted he was in bed by 10 p.m. on the night in question. It was noted that Hay had irregularities in his upper incisor teeth which prompted the question whether he would agree to have dental impressions taken to compare with the bite marks on the murder victim. The procedure adopted was to take each of twenty-nine boys in turn to Glasgow Dental Hospital to have casts made of their teeth. Each boy was designated by a number so that Dr Harvey would not know their identity when he compared the impressions with the crime scene evidence. It was at this point that he called on Keith Simpson for assistance, acknowledging the need for additional expertise.

Comparing the casts with photographs of the bite marks, attention was drawn to Number 14 as the most likely match, although Dr Harvey did not think the identification was sufficiently strong to precipitate the arrest of a suspect. Having narrowed the field to five of the plaster casts, Simpson and Harvey adopted a different strategy. They made models in acrylic material and hinged the two halves so that they could simulate a bite. Then, as Simpson later described it in his matter-of-fact way, as soon as a suitable female body appeared during the normal course of mortuary work, we 'made trial marks on the breast'. The advantage of the odontologist and the pathologist combining their efforts was immediately apparent, with the effect that cast Number 14 was eliminated.

It was back to the drawing board, and the two experts began to concentrate on two small pits visible in the bite mark impression left on the victim, which had been previously noted. Dr Harvey had not come across any references to features such as these in the scientific literature and acknowledged that they were now in unchartered waters. Reviewing all the casts once more with this particular feature in mind, their focus came to rest on Cast Number 11 which showed a damaged upper incisor and another tooth with a small cavity due to a missing filling. There was a perfect match with the bite impression on the victim.

Elated, yet cautious, they discussed their dental investigation, which had taken several weeks to complete, with Chief Superintendent Muncie. He confirmed that from other circumstantial evidence gleaned from the scene of the crime, Number 11 was also his suspect. Yet the experts had some lingering doubts. Forensic odontology was still in its relative infancy and the textbook marker for dental identification was a minimum of four or five adjacent teeth – Harvey and Simpson only had three. So, once again, it was back to the drawing board.

Further impressions were taken of Number 11's teeth and subjected to intense scrutiny by Dr Harvey. Transparencies made from them were superimposed on photographs of the bite marks and examined by Keith Simpson. His opinion was that the results were like matching fingerprints. This was sufficient corroboration of identity to prompt the issue of a warrant to arrest Gordon Hay and, in due course, he appeared on trial for the murder of Linda Peacock. Simpson gave evidence and said that in more than thirty years, 'I have not seen a bite mark with better defined detail than this.' Dr Harvey's evidence took a full day to deliver. Simpson described him as the prosecution's 'star witness'. His meticulous preparation was apparent to the extent that he had examined the dentition of over 300 youths and found only two with a pit on the tip of a canine tooth.

Hay gave evidence which consisted mostly of denials and his defence counsel was at pains to stress that the Crown's evidence was circumstantial. In his summing up, the judge referred to forensic dentistry as, 'a relatively new science', while emphasising that the law must keep pace with science. The jury took two and a half hours to consider their verdict. They pronounced the defendant guilty and he was ordered to be detained during Her Majesty's Pleasure. An appeal was lodged and dismissed, leaving William Muncie to record in his memoirs, *The Crime Pond*, published in 1979, that 'a case, unique in British criminal annals' was concluded.

Pathologists do not like loose ends and unsolved murders certainly fall into that category. Despite many confessions and accusations, all of them false, the murder of Joan Woodhouse in 1948 remains unsolved. The twenty-seven-year-old librarian from Yorkshire was found dead in Arundel Park, Sussex in circumstances which offered conflicting interpretations. What was inescapable, though, was that the young woman had been raped and strangled. Her partially-clothed body was found on 10 August by Thomas Stilwell, an Arundel man, while walking through the park. The body lay on sloping ground in a copse away from regularly used pathways. The dead woman was lying on her back, dressed in her underwear with no apparent attempts at concealment. Her outer clothes, together with a necklace and handbag, lay neatly folded and placed nearby.

Keith Simpson carried out a post-mortem examination on the maggot-strewn corpse which he estimated had lain where it was found for eight to ten days. Looking at the bruises on the head and neck, he thought that she had been forced down by her assailant while he applied a strangling grip around her neck. The hyoid bone was fractured and the lungs and heart showed evidence of asphyxia. The dead woman's panties were still in place, although the pathologist determined that she had been subjected to forceful sexual intercourse. There were also signs of bruising on her thighs and around the vagina. Curiously, he found a ball of pubic hair in the vagina which he took as a further indication of the rough nature of the sexual assault that had occurred. The soft tissues had been broken down by the activity of maggots, making it impossible to swab for semen.

Chief Inspector Fred Narborough of Scotland Yard met Simpson at Arundel to review the crime scene. They had worked together before and the policeman was somewhat in awe of the pathologist whom he referred to as, 'That remarkable man'. They viewed the body as it lay under beech trees in a secluded area of the park. As the doctor went about his work, Narborough said later, '. . . my eyes kept returning to that neat pile of clothing – so neat and tidy – so carefully arranged.' It was a vision that haunted him to the end of his career.

A great deal was learned about Joan Woodhouse's background. She was an only child brought up in a highly religious Yorkshire family. She qualified as a librarian in London, taught in Sunday school and lived in the YMCA at Blackheath. It was known that she had met and fallen in love with an ex-serviceman and her friends saw her as a bright, happy person with a possible engagement in the offing. But, at Eastertime in 1948, her mood changed when it seemed the relationship with her intended fiancé broke down. He, apparently, did not share her High Church beliefs and a rift developed between them. Such was her unhappiness, that, in April, she tried to kill herself by overdosing on sleeping tablets. Those who knew her felt her personality had changed and she told a friend in July that she planned to visit her family in Yorkshire over the Bank Holiday weekend. Instead, she took a train to Worthing in Sussex and then travelled by bus to Arundel where she was last seen at around 2 p.m. on 31 July. When she failed to turn up for work after the weekend, she was reported missing and her body was found just over a week later.

Chief Inspector Narborough and Keith Simpson tried to work out what had happened on that fateful sunny day in Arundel Park. There were at least two possible scenarios. The first was that she had a secret assignation with the man who had until recently been her fiancé and that things had become argumentative and got out of hand. The second proposition, based on information given to the police by the dead woman's family, was that she was an ardent sun-worshipper who used every opportunity to sunbathe. This opened up the possibility that she went to a secluded section of the park, partially stripped off to lie in the sun and was surprised by a passing man who thought she might be inviting sexual liaison. Presented with an opportunity, he forced himself on her with violent consequences. In all the discussions, Fred Narborough's mind kept going back to that pile of neatly stacked clothes.

The detective set out to interview every friend and acquaintance of the dead woman in order to eliminate them from his enquiries. He also had three confessions to contend with from publicity-seeking individuals and wasters of police time. Joan Woodhouse's ex-fiancé was quickly eliminated from the enquiry when he was shown to have a sound and fully corroborated alibi. The inquest, held on 22 November 1948, concluded that the young woman had been murdered by a person or persons unknown. Dissatisfied with this outcome, her grieving family hired a private detective to search for the murderer. As a result, a report was sent to Scotland Yard naming as a suspect the man who had found her body in Arundel Park.

The Director of Public Prosecutions gave it as his opinion that there was insufficient evidence on which to base any meaningful prosecution. Undeterred by this apparent setback, Woodhouse's father applied to magistrates for a warrant to arrest the man in an attempted private prosecution. This was the first time such an application had been made in eighty-five years and it prompted a hearing at Arundel in September 1950 when the magistrates ruled there was no case to answer. Thus the family's hope of finding closure over Joan Woodhouse's death petered out.

In a subsequent development, Scotland Yard decided to re-open the investigation under the leadership of Detective Superintendent Reginald Spooner, as Fred Narborough had, by then, retired. Keith Simpson expressed surprise at the turn of events and, particularly as Spooner did not consult him before launching his own theory regarding Joan Woodhouse's death. The detective's view was that the young librarian had not been raped or even murdered, but had committed suicide. The pathologist thought this was an absurd notion. After all, he had clearly established that a sexual assault had taken place and that the victim had been strangled. His view was that Joan Woodhouse had been raped at the spot where her clothes lay neatly folded, a mute testimony to her relaxed frame of mind, and that she attempted to run away, only to be pursued by her attacker, who killed her. She was left for dead under the shelter of trees about thirty feet away.

Of all the theories, once the main suspects had been eliminated, was Keith Simpson's reconstruction based on his post-mortem findings. Joan Woodhouse, possibly in a disturbed state of mind following the break-up with her boyfriend, wanted to get away from it all and simply relax by soaking up the sun. Thinking she was safe in a secluded, wooded corner of Arundel Park, she took off her outer clothing and stretched out on the grass with the sun on her face. Her misfortune was to be seen by someone, a passing opportunist, who saw the possibility of a lustful adventure. When she ran off after he sexually assaulted her, he gave chase and silenced her before she could call for help. Perhaps the last word, quite literally, on this unsolved murder, should rest with Fred Narborough. His book of memoirs published in 1959, concluded with the line, 'All the time, there is that murder on my mind.'

A pathologist's repertoire of cases would not be complete without a few poisonings. They make a change from the round of fatal shootings, stabbings and strangulations and are often more imaginative than other forms of killing. Poisoning usually involves careful premeditation and calls for subtlety, stealth and cunning. Keith Simpson had his quota of poison cases and often shared their investigation with his old sparring partner, Francis Camps. A number of these are described in Chapter Four but one which stands out in Simpson's archives is a case which he described as 'one of the coolest murders by arsenic that ever came to lie in my crime files ...'. Margery Radford was very ill with pulmonary tuberculosis and was being treated at Milford Sanatorium at Godalming, Surrey. She was pale and very thin and relied on relatives to bring her food and drinks to stimulate her jaded appetite. Her husband, Frederick, was an attentive visitor, invariably bringing her fruit and soft drinks. He worked as a laboratory technician at nearby St Thomas's Hospital.

These bedside rituals were dramatically interrupted one day in April 1949 when Mrs Radford experienced constant vomiting after eating a fruit pie which her husband had given to a relative to take to her. She confided in a friend, Mrs Formby, who visited her in the sanatorium saying she believed that she was being poisoned as a result of eating some of the things brought in by her husband. She asked her friend if she would send the fruit pie to Scotland Yard for analysis. This was an unusual request and her friend responded not by contacting the police, but by leaving the pie in the office of the sanatorium superintendent with a note saying a letter of explanation would follow. This was a course of action that was to have a dramatic outcome.

Unaware of the significance attached to the pie, the Superintendent took it home with the thought that some well-meaning visitor had left him a little treat. He took a few bites out of the pie and quickly became unwell with violent stomach pains and severe vomiting. He spent the remainder of the weekend in bed recovering from his sickness and wondering about the provenance of the fruit pie. He returned to work on Monday where Mrs Formby's letter voicing Margery Radford's concerns was waiting on his desk. He showed the remainder of the pie to Mrs Radford who identified it.

The police were informed of the turn of events and arranged for the offending pie's contents to be analysed at Scotland Yard's laboratory. The analyst found over 3 grains of potassium arsenite in the pie and immediately reported his discovery to detectives. On the same day, 12 April 1949, Margery Radford died. Keith Simpson carried out the post-mortem examination supported by Scotland Yard's analyst. He confirmed the advanced state of the dead woman's tuberculosis and found that her frail body was riddled with poison. From the arsenic present in her hair roots it was possible to estimate that she had been systematically poisoned over a period of twelve weeks. As the pathologist observed, Margery Radford's deterioration was put down to her tuberculosis and none of the medical staff at the sanatorium suspected, or had any reason to suspect, that she was also being poisoned.

When he was interviewed by detectives, Frederick Radford asked, 'Why should I want to kill my wife? I knew she was going to die anyway.' He pointed out that as a laboratory technician he knew how easy it was to detect arsenic and would not have been so foolish to use it. He challenged the police to charge him and let the jury decide the outcome. He attended the opening of the inquest into his wife's death and was driven home afterwards in a police car. Keith Simpson said in his memoirs that Radford invited the officers into his home for a cup of tea but, as he put it, 'they understandably declined.' On the following day, Radford was found dead in bed, having taken his own life with poison. He knew that arsenic was for the long haul so he chose cyanide as the fastest means of procuring his own death.

But for Margery Radford's suspicions, it is likely that her own death would have been recorded as due to the tuberculosis from which she was suffering and her husband would have got away with murder. The assumption was that Radford grew tired of looking after his chronically sick wife and decided to assist her departure from a tormented life.

Simpson noted that general medical practitioners as a rule do not include the possibility of murder in their considerations of cause of death. The symptoms of poisoning may masquerade as genuine illness and the sick bed environment of the chronically ill provides ready cover for the intending poisoner, as in the case of Frederick Radford. Writing in 1972, Keith Simpson noted that only 0.2 per cent of all deaths from poison were attributable to arsenic.

Determining the distinction between accident, murder and suicide is among the judgements a pathologist makes on a daily basis and it is not always straightforward. In 1959, Simpson managed to solve the riddle of two deaths in Portugal despite having been prevented from examining the circumstances at first hand. In February of that year, a family of four set out from England for a motoring holiday in Portugal which ended tragically when Arthur and Patricia Trist were found dead in their motel chalet, leaving their two children as survivors. The family had settled into their accommodation near Lisbon and, after putting the two children to bed, the couple went out for a meal. The alarm was raised the next day when the maid reported that after three attempts, she had failed to get a response from the occupants of the chalet. The manager decided to force the door and found Arthur and Patricia dead and two very confused children who could not get their parents to wake up. Police were called to the scene but found nothing that might indicate foul play.

The two bodies were examined by a local police surgeon who found no injuries on either. The knowledge that the dead couple had dined out on shell food the previous evening, linked to vomit stains on their clothing, led the Portuguese authorities to conclude that the cause of death was food poisoning. This diagnosis did not hold up too well when enquiries showed that other diners at the restaurant who had also eaten shell fish suffered no ill-effects. Nevertheless, the authorities were adamant that the cause of death of the two English visitors was food poisoning. Requests that a pathologist from Britain should be allowed to examine the bodies were indignantly refused.

By this time, Keith Simpson had been asked to review the post-mortem findings and he quickly identified several shortcomings. The poor quality of the examination carried out by local doctors was highlighted when their report mentioned the condition of both lungs in Patricia Trist's body. As her medical records confirmed, she only had one lung following surgery several years earlier. Simpson noted that blood and muscle samples needed to test for carbon monoxide poisoning had not been taken. This was especially significant in view of reports from representatives of the family who had been permitted to enter the chalet and take stock of the surroundings in which the Trists had died. Their attention focussed on the bathroom which was very small and fitted with a gas water heater. The ventilation was poor and there was no flue to conduct combustion fumes to the outside of the building.

The pathologist suspected carbon monoxide poisoning was the likely cause of death and the indications of vomiting were consistent with this. These conclusions were put to the Portuguese authorities but were promptly rejected on the grounds that the matter had already been resolved. The importance of establishing an accurate cause of death lay in any claims made by the two surviving children of the tragedy and the accident insurance which had been taken out by their father. Having been denied the opportunity to carry out independent post-mortem examinations, Simpson played what he later described as his 'trump card'. The Trist family's request to the Portuguese for the return of the bodies to their homeland could hardly be refused and was duly acted upon. As soon as he viewed the returned corpses in his laboratory at Guy's Hospital and saw the tell-tale cherry-pink colour of their skin, he knew that carbon monoxide poisoning was the cause of their deaths. The mystery, as he later described it, was that the Portuguese medical examiners had missed the obvious.

The source of the carbon monoxide was the gas water heater in the holiday chalet which subsequent tests showed was of a type that could build up a fatal concentration of gas in a confined and ill-ventilated space. The Portuguese authorities were notified of these latest findings but continued to hold firm to their original line that the English couple had died of food poisoning. The family's insurance company honoured the policy which Arthur Trist had taken out before the ill-fated family holiday.

There was some diplomatic fall-out following this case, when Portugal complained to the Foreign Office about the British pathologist's involvement in the enquiry. This was to rebound some twenty years later with headlines in the British press about deaths in the Algarve from carbon monoxide poisoning arising from faulty gas water heaters. The *Sunday Times*, on 23 January 1983, reported the deaths of ten British tourists in Portugal holiday resorts, claiming that death certificates were issued with incorrect causes of death, including natural causes and food poisoning, when the classic indications of carbon monoxide poisoning evident on post-mortem examination should have alerted local doctors to the real cause. Interviewed by the newspaper, Professor Simpson was quoted as saying, 'It's disgraceful' and observing that the cases discovered were 'the tip of the iceberg'. The press reports provoked concerns about the safety of British tourists and raised questions regarding the quality of Portuguese investigation of unexpected deaths.

Some murder cases, although apparently closed, seem to rumble on in the public conscience for years. One such was the A6 Murder, for which James Hanratty was judged guilty and hanged. Keith Simpson was called to the scene of a fatal shooting on a stretch of road known as Deadman's Hill on 23 August 1961. A double shooting had occurred in the early hours of the morning which left Michael Gregston dead and his lover, Valerie Storie, badly wounded. The couple had been sitting in their parked car near Slough when they were threatened by a man with a gun. He sat in the rear seat and ordered them to drive away. After travelling north for about thirty miles, he told Gregston to pull into a lay-by on the A6.

There, he shot Gregston twice in the head and, after raping Valerie Storie, fired five shots at her, leaving her paralysed. The assailant then drove away in their car.

Keith Simpson examined Gregston's body at Bedford Mortuary, confirming that he had died between 3 and 4 a.m. from gunshot wounds consisting of two .32 calibre shots fired at close range. A few days later, he visited Valerie Storie in hospital and examined her wounds, five in all, also from a .32 weapon. He found her remarkably clear and lucid in the account she gave of the incident which he found entirely consistent with the medical evidence. Although badly injured, Storie was able to describe the gunman to the police and an Identikit picture was published seeking information from the public. This was followed by a second Identikit based on a description of a man seen driving Gregston's car which was later found abandoned. The murder weapon was found on a London bus and two cartridge cases linked to it were discovered in a London hotel room that had been occupied on the night before the murder by James Hanratty using an alias. On the night of the murder, the room was occupied by Peter Alphon, a commercial traveller.

Hanratty was arrested in Blackpool on 9 October and, despite his lack of resemblance to either of the Identikit pictures, was identified as the A6 gunman. He claimed an alibi which placed him in Liverpool at the crucial time but, later, changed his story. He was charged with murder and subsequently found guilty. Hanratty was hanged on 4 April 1962, but public disquiet prompted the Home Office to re-open the case in 1967 after Alphon made a confession, claiming he had been asked to end the relationship between Gregston and Storie. The idea was to frighten the couple but the gun discharged accidentally and Hanratty was framed for the murder.

Simpson was in no doubt about the validity of the original verdict which he said had not been shaken by subsequent claims. This was borne out by events in 2002 when the case went to the Court of Appeal. Hanratty's body had been exhumed in order to obtain a DNA sample that could be compared with DNA found on garments relating to the case which had previously been mislaid. The results of these tests ruled out Alphon as a suspect and the appeal judges upheld the original conviction of James Hanratty.

When, in a social context, Keith Simpson might be asked what was currently engaging his attention, he would often reply, 'Oh! You know, scribble, scribble.' As much as he enjoyed lecturing, he also liked putting pen to paper. This was evident early in his career when he wrote his textbook, *Forensic Medicine*, first published in 1947. It ran to many editions and earned an accolade from *The Criminologist* for containing '. . . a phenomenal range of knowledge and information'. In 1958, the book won professional recognition when the Royal Society of Arts awarded it the Swiney Prize. After Sir Sydney Smith's retirement, Simpson took on the editorship of *Taylor's Principles and Practice of Medical Jurisprudence*. This was a prodigious task, refreshing and updating a textbook regarded by many as the bible of the forensic practitioner. Alfred Swaine Taylor first published the book in 1836 and it has run to many editions since. Professor Simpson also wrote what was, arguably, the first textbook intended for crime scene investigators. *Police: The Investigation of Violence*, published in 1978, was written in forthright language and used explicit illustrations. The book was well received by police training establishments. He also found time to write novels and other books using the pseudonym Guy Bailey. *The Fatal Chance*, published in 1969, included a number of his cases such as Haigh and Sangret, in which chance played a major role in crime investigation.

Estimating time of death is a constant challenge for the forensic pathologist with many environmental factors to be taken into consideration. It is made to look easy in televised crime dramas but, in practice, requires a great deal of skill and experience. Occasionally, nature gives a helping hand and such was the case when two boys went out searching in Bracknell Woods, Berkshire for maggots to use as fish bait. Their practice was to find an animal carcass from which they could retrieve a few maggots as it decomposed and the flesh provided a breeding ground for bluebottle flies.

On 28 June 1964, the two lads found a treasure trove of heaving maggots on a mound of earth and leaves. But, as they began retrieving the larvae to put in their collecting jars, they uncovered a human forearm and lost no time in reporting their discovery to the police. A telephone call to Professor Simpson was not long delayed and he was quickly at the scene. His first task was carefully to disinter the body of which the exposed forearm was the only visible part. He found the corpse of a fully-clothed man, lying face uppermost with a towel wrapped around the head.

The pathologist knew it was a waste of time taking body temperatures in view of the extent of decomposition and realised that the maggots represented the best chance of establishing how long the man had been dead. One of the police officers observing Simpson at work suggested the body had been dead for six or eight weeks and was astonished when the pathologist told him that it was more likely to have been nine or ten days. He picked off some of the maggots which he thought were a species of bluebottle and put them into a specimen jar for later study. The maggots were third-stage larvae hatched from eggs which he estimated had been laid nine or ten days previously. By adding extra time, allowing for the flies to seek out the corpse, Simpson calculated that death had occurred around 16 or 17 June.

Examining the rotting remains of the head and neck *in situ*, Simpson found that the bones of the larynx were broken on the left side, indicating some kind of blow to the throat. Later, in the mortuary, he found signs of asphyxia in the heart muscle and there was blood in the windpipe. His conclusion, in the absence of any other indicators, was that the injuries to the man's throat had led to inhalation of blood with death ensuing very quickly. The height of the body was calculated at five feet three inches and X-rays showed a mended fracture of the left forearm. Fingerprints were obtained from the decomposing skin left on the hands which unequivocally identified the dead man as Peter Thomas, an individual whose fingerprints were in police records. CID officers had been combing through missing persons files and established that forty-two-year-old Thomas had disappeared from his home in Gloucestershire on 16 June.

Detectives from the West Country now put their heads together with colleagues from Berkshire to consider how and why Peter Thomas's body had ended up in woodlands a hundred miles from his home. It seemed that he lived alone with only his dog as a companion in a dilapidated bungalow at Lydney. His day-to-day existence depended on social welfare payments. A search of his home turned up a letter referring to a loan of £2,000 which had been made to one William Brittle, and which was due to be repaid in mid-June. Brittle, a salesman for heating systems, lived at Hook in Hampshire. When interviewed by detectives, he said he had driven to Lydney to see Thomas in order to repay the loan. To corroborate his story, he said he had given a lift to a hitch-hiker on his return journey to Hampshire. This individual was traced by the police and he confirmed that Brittle had indeed given him a lift.

Meanwhile forensic technicians were taking a close look at Brittle's car but found nothing of significance. The enquiry was beginning to run out of steam when a man came forward with the information that he had seen Peter Thomas, a former acquaintance, at Gloucester bus station on 20 June, four days after he was presumed to be dead. This obviously jeopardised the case the police were building up against William Brittle, but Simpson stuck to his original estimate that death had occurred on 16 or 17 June. There was some vacillation in high places and the Director of Public Prosecutions decided the evidence against Brittle was insufficiently strong to warrant a trial.

Although they may have been disappointed by this turn of events, the Gloucestershire police decided on a different strategy and referred the case against Brittle to the coroner at Bracknell in Berkshire. The inquest jury's verdict there was that Peter Thomas had been murdered and Brittle was named as the perpetrator. To the surprise of the medico-legal fraternity, the coroner's jury had gone against the ruling made earlier by the Director of Public Prosecutions and Brittle was committed to stand trial. He was due to appear at the Spring Assizes in Gloucester in 1965. The defence team called on Dr David Bowen, a colleague

of Donald Teare at St George's Hospital, to advise them and also a leading entomologist, Professor McKenny-Hughes. During the trial, the prosecutor, Ralph
Cusack QC, argued that Brittle had murdered Peter Thomas, put his body in
his car boot and driven from Gloucestershire to Berkshire where he buried it in
woods near Bracknell. His motive was to be rid of a creditor who was pressing
him for repayment of a loan.

There was general agreement that Thomas had died following a blow to the
throat which caused haemorrhaging into the air passages and led to death by
asphyxia. The nature of the blow to the throat had echoes of the Emmett-Dunne
case twelve years earlier when a senior army NCO was found to have killed a
fellow Sergeant with a chopping blow to the throat and then faked his suicide.
The pathologist involved at the time was Francis Camps, Simpson's old adversary,
who, quite possibly, was reading the press reports about the trial at Gloucester
with special interest. In the course of their enquiries, the police learned that
Brittle had served in the army and attended a course where he was trained in the
use of unarmed combat techniques. He had been discharged from the service for
passing himself off as an officer.

The proceedings against Brittle hinged on the behaviour of maggots. The father
of forensic entomology was Professor Jean-Pierre Mégnin, a French military vet-
erinarian. He published his research on the life cycle of blowflies in 1894 and
showed that insect activity on a corpse could provide accurate indications of the
post-mortem interval. He thereby established the foundations of modern forensic
entomology. The larvae in question at Brittle's trial were *Calliphora erythrocephalus*
hatched from eggs laid by bluebottle flies. Eggs are customarily laid in warm
weather in daylight hours and hatch out on the same day. The first development
(instar) occurs after eight to fourteen hours, the second instar (two to three days)
and the third, fully grown instar, after five to six days, before the maggot pupates
with a hard shell. Hence, as estimated by Keith Simpson, making an allowance for
the flies to find the body, some eleven to twelve days might have elapsed, thereby
placing Thomas's death on 16 or 17 June.

Simpson gave his evidence, supported by sketches he had made at the scene
and by photographs. Next came Professor McKenny-Hughes, who had seen
the maggots which the pathologist had taken as specimens from the body in
the woods and confirmed that they were indeed larvae of the bluebottle. Asked
how his views on the habits and life cycle differed from Simpson's, the professor
declined to criticise his colleague, so, moving swiftly on, the prosecutor, Quinton
Hogg QC, posed a theoretical question as to what might result when, '. . . the
bluebottle lays its eggs on the dead body at midnight . . .'. The professor recoiled
in horror at the thought and replied, 'No self-respecting bluebottle lays eggs at
midnight.' The sniggers around the court heralded a triumph for Keith Simpson
whose evidence regarding time of death was accepted by the jury in preference

to the evidence of the witness who claimed to have seen Peter Thomas after he was presumed to be dead. The pathologist had won the day and expressed pleasure that his reputation for calculating time of death had been vindicated. The trial jury found William Brittle guilty and he was sentenced to life imprisonment.

To his busy lecturing and writing schedules, Simpson also added an international dimension. His reputation as a painstaking and reliable forensic examiner resulted in invitations to visit other countries to train crime scene investigators and also to assist in murder enquiries. His visit to Canada in 1967 to give evidence at the re-trial of Steven Truscott gave him satisfaction over Francis Camps at the time when the judgement given confirmed the original verdict of Truscott's guilt. The full story is told in Chapter Four and serves as an example of the precept held by forensic pathologists that things are not always as they seem. Whereas, in 1967, Simpson's opinion was at odds with that of Camps, the passage of forty years would reverse the earlier affirmation of Truscott's guilt and confirm his innocence. He was paroled in 1969 having been sentenced to death ten years earlier. Fearful of its image as a fair-minded country, the Canadian Government had commuted the death sentence passed on the fourteen-year-old boy. In 2008, Truscott was cleared of all allegations and offered substantial compensation. By then, both Camps and Simpson, arch rivals on the forensic scene, had buried their differences to the extent that both had passed on.

Keith Simpson joined the international forensic circuit in the early 1970s and made numerous trips in the role of lecturer and adviser. He undertook several visits to the West Indies and, notably, to Trinidad in 1972, at the request of the British Foreign Office. There was great excitement, not to say, anxiety, in Port of Spain when he arrived poste haste from London. On 19 February the fire brigade had been called out to attend a blaze at *La Chance*, the home of Abdul Malik, also known as Michael X, a controversial figure in the Black Power movement. The house was completely destroyed in the fire and when the police arrived at the scene and searched the grounds, an observant officer noticed that a bed of lettuce in the garden was unusually luxuriant with tall, yellow plants sprouting out of it. The lettuce was probed and found to be masking a grave which contained a man's body. Further digging in the garden two days later revealed the discovery of a second grave containing a female corpse.

The background to these grim discoveries was the influence which Abdul Malik exerted over a band of devoted followers based at *La Chance* and living as a commune. Born in Trinidad as Michael de Freitas, he adopted the Muslim faith in 1963 and changed his name. He was active in London's immigrant communities in the mid-1960s and founded the Racial Advancement Action Society.

Firmly under the influence of Malcolm X, the American Black Power leader, he returned to Trinidad in 1969 where he fomented strife, preaching a brand of extreme racialism which brought him into conflict with the law. He threatened to deal with the 'white monkeys' and talked of killing with a clear conscience. His ambition to influence religious and political groups did not succeed, despite his claims, although he continued to exert control over his close band of followers.

In the aftermath of the fire at *La Chance*, Malik disappeared, leaving the police and pathologists to find explanations for what had happened there. The dead woman was identified as Gail Benson, a twenty-year-old English girl, one of Malik's followers, who, it was estimated, had been dead for about two months. She had been attacked with a knife and sustained several wounds including a deep thrust through her neck which penetrated into her chest. Disturbingly, Keith Simpson discovered evidence suggesting that the victim had not been dead when her body was put into the ground and covered with soil. He found particles of earth in her throat and air passages, indicating that she was still breathing when interred. There was also evidence that she had put up a struggle, although there was no indication of any sexual assault.

The second body, buried in the lettuce patch, was that of Joe Skerrit, Malik's cousin, who functioned as handyman at *La Chance*. He had been decapitated with a cutlass and buried in the garden. It emerged later that both killings had been carried out on Malik's instructions; Gail Benson because she was not sufficiently compliant with his wishes, and Skerrit, who simply refused to obey the orders he was given. By these means, Malik sought to maintain control over his followers. Meanwhile, he had absconded to Guyana, ostensibly on a lecture tour. He was located by the authorities and deported to Trinidad where he faced murder charges.

The full extent of his evil influence came out during his trial at Port of Spain's Assize Court in January 1972. Simpson attended to give evidence amid tight security, for there were fears that Malik might stage some kind of demonstration. The pathologist was chaperoned by plain-clothes officers as he prepared to go into court. His testimony was not contested and was amply supported by witnesses who described the circumstances under which Benson and Skerrit met violent deaths under a tropical sun. The proceedings did provide him with at least one humorous interlude when a local expert professed to be able to distinguish human from animal blood just by looking at it. Counsel said, 'If you can do that, you must be a genius. Are you a genius?' to which the witness replied simply, 'Yes.' This was a perfect example of the legal precept that lawyers should not ask questions to which they do not already know the answer.

Malik was convicted of murder and one of his accomplices was found guilty of manslaughter. The following year, two more members of Malik's malign group were convicted of murdering Gail Benson. His appeal against sentence of death was turned down by the Privy Council in London and he was executed on

16 May 1975. Of Malik's unhappy band of followers, two were murdered, one died accidentally and two were hanged.

As his international reputation grew, so Keith Simpson found that he had a fuller than ever in-tray. Letters came to him from all corners of the globe seeking information and asking for opinions. Occasionally they bore exotic forms of address such as Professor of Scenic Medicine or, more suggestively, Professor of Foreskinic Medicine.

Closer to home, Keith Simpson was drawn in to one of the twentieth century's great mysteries – the Lord Lucan affair. Late in the evening of 7 November 1974, a distraught woman, bleeding from a head wound, burst into The Plumber's Arms public house in lower Belgrave Street in London's West End. She called for help between sobs and screamed, 'I have just escaped from a murder!' She feared for her children and shouted, 'He's in the house . . . He's murdered the nanny . . . Help me!' This dramatic outburst was the overture to what would become known as 'The Lord Lucan Affair', which, nearly forty years later, still retains its essential mystery – the whereabouts of Lord Lucan, dead or alive.

The injured woman who had so startled the customers at The Plumber's Arms was Lady Lucan. While the pub landlady sought to calm her, calls were made to the ambulance service and the police. Lady Lucan was taken to hospital and, soon afterwards, two police officers arrived at the pub before going on to the Lucan family home at 46 Lower Belgrave Street. The door of the house was locked and the officers had to force an entry to the premises which were in complete darkness. They found bloodstains on the wall in the hallway and a pool of blood at the bottom of the stairs leading down to the basement. They checked the rooms in other parts of the house and found three children, two asleep and one watching television.

Returning to the basement where there was a breakfast room, they saw a canvas mailbag with an arm protruding from it. Inside the bag was the still warm, doubled-up body of Sandra Rivett, the Lucan's nanny. She was dead from head injuries assumed to have been inflicted with a length of bloodstained lead pipe found later in the hallway. The police surgeon pronounced life extinct and the body was taken to the mortuary where, next morning, Keith Simpson carried out a post-mortem examination. The pathologist determined that death had been caused by several blunt force injuries to the head. While the skull was not fractured, he found bruising and haemorrhaging in the brain. Both of the dead woman's shoulders were heavily bruised and there was what Simpson described as 'protective' bruising on the back of her right hand. He judged that bruising evident on the upper arm had resulted from being forcefully gripped and believed she was dead before being bundled up and put into the mailbag.

He found that there had been copious bleeding from the head injuries into the throat and air passages and, due to the fact that she was only semi-conscious, would have been unable to clear her airways with the result that she died within minutes. Shown the piece of bloodstained lead piping by detectives, Simpson believed it could have been used to inflict the injuries he had described. Lady Lucan had also been attacked and injured by an assailant, probably using the same bludgeoning instrument. The piece of pipe weighed 2¼lb and had surgical tape wrapped around it.

Having being patched up in hospital and re-assured that her children were safe, Lady Lucan gave the police an account of what had taken place at 46 Lower Belgrave Street. She said that she and her ten-year-old daughter were watching television in the bedroom and Sandra Rivett went down to the basement kitchen to make tea just before 9 p.m. When the nanny had not re-emerged by 9.15 and while the television news was being broadcast, Lady Lucan went downstairs to find out the reason for the delay.

The basement was in darkness and there was no response when she called out Sandra's name. Then she heard a noise and someone attacked her with a heavy object, striking her on the head. She was told to 'shut up' and recognised the voice as her husband's. She struggled with him and he handled her roughly before seeming to calm down and then they both moved upstairs to the bedroom. While Lucan went into the bathroom to fetch a towel to mop up the blood on her face, Lady Lucan fled from the house, out into the street and headed for The Plumber's Arms. At this point, Lord Lucan disappeared, thereby creating an enduring crime mystery.

The inquest into Sandra Rivett's death opened in June 1975 at Westminster coroner's court under the direction of Dr Gavin Thurston. A great deal of the proceedings was taken up by testimony relating to Lord and Lady Lucan's relationship and family background. Richard John Bingham attended Eton and became an officer in the Coldstream Guards. He married Veronica in 1963 and, in the following year, succeeded to the title of Seventh Earl of Lucan. He moved in elite social circles and acquired a reputation as a gambler for which he was nicknamed 'Lucky Lucan'. He was accustomed to winning or losing as much as £5,000 a day. The Lucans' marriage broke up in 1974 and Veronica took custody of the three children. She continued to live in the house in Lower Belgrave Street.

In the immediate aftermath of the violent incident which took place on 7 November, Lucan fled the scene and later telephoned his mother to tell her he had found an intruder attacking his wife. Late on the night of Sandra Rivett's death, he visited a friend in East Sussex to whom he explained that his wife had accused him of hiring someone to kill her. Two days later, Lucan wrote to another friend saying that he intended to lie low. His car was found the next day near Newhaven, its interior stained with blood and a piece of lead piping found in the boot. The blood traces tested positive for both A and B groups and also AB.

The dead woman was Group B (8.5 per cent of the population) and Lady Lucan Group A (42 per cent of the population).

The lead pipe found in the abandoned car was from the same length of piping found at the scene of the attack and had been similarly wrapped with surgical tape. Fingerprints found at the house were all accounted for, implying that the attacker, if he were a stranger, left no prints. The inquest jury's verdict was that Sandra Rivett had been murdered by Lord Lucan. The law whereby a coroner's court could name a murderer in this way was abolished following this case and the introduction of The Criminal Law Act in 1977. But, in 1975, Lord Lucan was named in his absence as a murderer and effectively judged as guilty.

Immense speculation ensued as to the whereabouts of Lord Lucan and sightings of him were reported all round the world. In 1987, two separate accounts of the killing of Sandra Rivett were published and both exonerated Lucan as the murderer. One theory was that he had hired a contract killer to eliminate his wife and the other suggested that the nanny had surprised a thief and paid for it with her life. While speculation continued, the central mystery remains – what happened to Lord Lucan? Keith Simpson concluded that the murderer had evidently gained entry using a house key and killed Rivett when she went down to the basement kitchen. As the police had not reported any indications of robbery, the pathologist believed that Rivett had been killed by mistake and that Lady Lucan was the real target. With the inquest verdict of 'Murder by Lord Lucan', Simpson quoted the Earl's words spoken to a friend on the night he disappeared; 'I don't want my children to see me standing in the dock.' As the pathologist put it rather drily in his memoirs, '. . . and they haven't'. That was written in 1978 and, thirty years later, they still haven't.

Perhaps, second only to the 'The Lucan Affair' in Keith Simpson's impressive collection of mysteries was the death of 'God's Banker'. Early on a summer's morning, 18 June 1982, a postman on his way to work walked under Blackfriars' Bridge in the City of London and saw a man's body dangling from a rope attached to a building maintenance scaffold. He had been suspended by his neck with a metre length of rope and his pockets were filled with stones and bricks weighing about five kilos. There was a passport bearing the name, Robert Calvini, in his pocket along with a wallet containing £7,000 in different currencies. The death of Robert Calvini, real name, Roberto Calvi, soon to be dubbed 'God's Banker' because of his connections with the Vatican, made big headlines in the media and the legal consequences of his dramatic death rumbled on for more than twenty years. It was far from being an open-and-shut case, although, from the outset, the police thought they were dealing with a straightforward hanging.

The body was taken to the City of London Mortuary where Keith Simpson carried out a post-mortem examination. He noted that the lower part of the trousers worn by the dead man were wet, whereas the upper clothing was merely damp.

A Patek Philippe watch on his wrist had stopped at 1.52 a.m. The man's age was estimated at around sixty-two and he weighed thirteen stone. The rope around his neck was loosely tied with a slip knot. The pathologist particularly noted a double groove on the skin marking a line on both sides of the neck and rising to a position at the back which he judged to be the point of suspension. The double indentation in the skin was probably due to the body being partially supported in water and the rope moving in response to changes in the level of the river. The view that this was a suicidal hanging tended to be confirmed by the presence of petechial haemorrhages in the eyelids, although there were no fractures in the larynx. Simpson thought the man had probably dropped about two feet before he hit the water, which accounted for the wet trousers. There were no indications of drowning.

The watch on the dead man's wrist was an obvious possible indicator of time of death insofar as it was not a waterproof model and might, therefore, have stopped when its owner's hands became submerged. The watery environment ruled out the usefulness of body temperature readings and rigor mortis was evident, although not complete. Taking all these factors into account, Keith Simpson thought that between eight and twelve hours had elapsed since death. Tide tables were another guide and showed that if hanging had occurred at around 2 a.m., the lower half of the body would have been immersed in the river during the night, before the tide receded to its lowest level, leaving the body clear of the water. This, combined with the other data, seemed to suggest that death occurred between 1 and 2.30 a.m.

Simpson gave evidence at the inquest held on 23 July and presided over by the City of London coroner, Dr David Paul, in what proved to be controversial proceedings. He testified that Calvi was, in all respects, a healthy individual in life. There was no disease of the brain and no evidence of any physical ailment that might have caused him any distress. He had found characteristic indications of asphyxia due to constriction of the neck, leading him to conclude that death was due to hanging. There were no marks on the body to suggest that any force had been applied and tests for alcohol and drugs were negative. 'There was,' the pathologist said, 'no evidence to suggest that the hanging was other than self-suspension . . .'.

The Calvi family was represented by Sir David Napley and the jury heard both written and oral testimony from forty witnesses. These included the foreman of the firm responsible for erecting the maintenance scaffold under Blackfriars' Bridge who said it would have been difficult for someone to carry a heavy weight down the access ladder to reach the scaffolding. The coroner summed up, listing the ways in which Calvi might have met his end. If he hanged himself, he either clambered down onto the scaffolding from the riverside or scrambled up onto it from a boat in the river. If he had been murdered, there was the question to be considered of his weight and the problems of negotiating a ladder and slippery scaffold planks if he had been lowered from above. Similar difficulties would have been encountered if his inert body had been delivered to the point of suspension by boat. Having considered the evidence, the jury returned a majority verdict of death by suicide. The response of the grieving widow was that her husband had been murdered and she said she would not rest until his killers were brought to justice. Sir David Napley made it known that an appeal would be lodged.

Enquiries into the background of Roberto Calvi's death revealed the complex inner workings of the international banking system. Many murky secrets came to the fore and several unsolved mysteries were highlighted. It seemed that God's Banker had close financial ties with the Vatican and, on the day before he died, he was stripped of his authority as head of Banco Ambrosiano. The bank crashed in 1982 with debts of £700m amid claims of false practices. These allegations had put Calvi under the spotlight in Italy where he faced charges of false accounting and exchange control violations. The inquest verdict in London did nothing to quell the rumours and Calvi's name was linked to that of Michele Sindona who had been convicted of fraud in the USA. Calvi's family believed he had been murdered to prevent him naming participants in the banking underworld.

On 29 March 1983, the Lord Chief Justice, Lord Lane, quashed the earlier suicide verdict and ordered a new enquiry because of irregularities in the way the first inquest was handled. Dr Paul was criticised because of statements he had made at the time. At the second inquest, under the direction of Dr Gordon Davies, the interests of the Calvi family were represented by George Carman QC. He pursued the angle that Roberto Calvi might have been rendered incapable of resistance due to the administration of an immobilising drug. This scenario would have enabled those who might wish to kill him to take his body by boat to the scaffolding platform under Blackfriars' Bridge in order to suspend it and, thereby, hang him.

An opposing theory was that Calvi, his pockets weighted with bricks, negotiated a twelve foot descent by ladder before stepping out onto the planking. Keith Simpson, cross-questioned by George Carman, said that when he examined the body, he ascertained that it had been immersed half-way up the legs. To counsel's suggestion that the body must have been wet, the pathologist replied that he assumed the body was in the position in which it was found. He mentioned that he had known situations where hanging was achieved from a sitting position. He would not change his original findings as to the cause of death but admitted the possibility that Calvi might have met his end at the hands of others. While the inquest jury was clear about the cause of death it was left with two possibilities as to the circumstances. The coroner said he saw no obvious evidence that the dead man had been unlawfully killed. On 27 June, the jury returned an open verdict.

During the following years, Calvi's name was rarely out of the news for one reason or another. The Prime Minister of Italy, Bettino Craxi, suggested in 1984 that the banker's death might have been linked to criminals operating within the banned P2 Masonic Lodge. And, in 1989, a court in Milan ruled that Calvi's death was murder. By this time, Keith Simpson had passed on, but the legacy of his work continued to produce new forensic challenges. In the same year, private investigators carried out a reconstruction of the tragedy at the request of the dead banker's son, Carlo Calvi. The original scaffolding from which the banker had been suspended had been kept in storage and the idea was to ask a stand-in to act the part of Calvi by climbing up on it. Examination of his shoes, similar to those worn by Calvi, carried traces of yellow paint and rust transferred to them from the metal scaffolding. No such traces had been found on the dead man's footwear in 1982, an observation which was used to reinforce the argument that he had not acted on his own account. This development was reported by Professor David Bowen in connection with an insurance claim relating to the case.

In June 1998, an Italian judge ordered that Calvi's body should be exhumed to establish whether his death was suicide or murder. There were hopes that finger-nail scrapings might still yield useful forensic material to help determine whether Calvi had handled the bricks used to weight his clothes. In July 2003, it was reported that Italian prosecutors had concluded Calvi was murdered and they suspected the involvement of four people. Their belief was that the banker had been killed by the Mafia for mishandling its money. The four men were put on trial in Rome in March 2004 when new evidence was introduced purporting to show that Calvi had been laundering treasury bonds stolen in 1982. In June 2007, a court in Rome decided there was insufficient evidence to convict the accused men and they secured an acquittal. The prosecution's case was that Calvi had been lured from his London apartment and was strangled before being taken by boat along the River Thames to Blackfriars' Bridge where his body was suspended from the scaffolding. This reconstruction of events was rejected by the judges.

More than twenty years after the discovery of a body under Blackfriars' Bridge, the mystery of Roberto Calvi's death remains. Commenting on the affair, Lico Gelli, the former Master of the P2 Masonic Lodge, was quoted as saying, 'It is not up to us to deliver judgements. Only God will be able to tell the truth.' Quite possibly, Keith Simpson would have agreed.

After his retirement in 1972 having served for twenty-six years at the Department of Forensic Medicine at London University, first as Reader and then as Professor, Keith Simpson was appointed Emeritus Professor and continued to lecture and examine at various universities, including Oxford, Cardiff and St Andrews. Despite all his accomplishments, perhaps the thing he regretted most was not being honoured with a knighthood. That would have given him parity with Spilsbury and Smith. He was awarded a CBE in 1978 and after being subsequently overlooked in the honours lists, he expressed his disappointment to Joe Gaute, his publisher, whose encouraging response was, 'Don't worry Keith, it will come.' Unfortunately, although thoroughly merited, it never did.

Apart from Francis Camps with whom he had a fractured relationship, Simpson achieved many plaudits from his contemporaries during his lifetime. Dr Ray Williams, Director of the Metropolitan Police Forensic Science Laboratory, said of him, 'He has a gift for the most lucid exposition of the subject I have ever heard,' adding, 'He is a real giant in his profession'. His gifts as a teacher and explainer were widely recognised and he noted a moment of quiet satisfaction in his memoirs, *Forty Years of Murder*. In 1970, after giving evidence at the Old Bailey, he was handed a note written to him by Leslie Boyd, the Senior Clerk to the court. It read, 'If I may respectfully say so, I still think you give evidence better than anyone else I know or can remember – and that includes Spilsbury.' The enjoyment of the comment was no doubt the greater for besting Spilsbury, at least in the Clerk's opinion.

Keith Simpson was, naturally, a member or fellow of many learned and distinguished clubs and societies but, perhaps, one of the least well known was Our Society, formerly The Crimes Club, a dining venue for medico-legal practitioners. Formed in 1903, the club had a formidable membership which included Sir Arthur Conan Doyle and Sir Bernard Spilsbury. Simpson's contemporaries, Francis Camps and Donald Teare, were also members. In 1979, he gave a memorable presentation of the Lydney Case which he entitled, 'A Riddle of Maggots'. It was not recorded whether any of the diners had to leave the table but the subject matter certainly called for strong stomachs.

Keith Simpson did not suffer fools gladly but he was generous to his friends. In 1982, he found time to write a foreword to *Murder Whatdunit* by Joe Gaute and Robin Odell. Joe was an old friend but in a book which set out to demystify forensic investigation for non-specialist readers, he might have viewed it as an over-simplification of a field in which he was, indisputably, a master. Instead, he wrote a very generous appraisal, describing the book as, 'an essential reference work for the crime writer and an accurate encyclopaedia of world history in the subject'. He was a perfectionist and as resolute in his opinions as was Spilsbury, for whom he had scant regard; '. . . he was a cold, aloof man. I never saw him laugh,' he said. Like many professionals in different fields, the pleasure in his work came from confronting a challenge and then finding answers. Of his discovery of the tell-tale gallstone when he searched through the acid-reduced remains of George Haigh's victim, he said, 'It was the most exciting moment I think I've ever had.'

Keith Simpson was the last of 'The Three Musketeers'; Francis Camps died in 1972 and Donald Teare in 1979. Simpson outlived them and died, aged seventy-eight, in 1985 from a brain tumour. With their passing, perhaps the golden age of the forensic pathologist also closed. The advances and reforms for which they had fought through teaching and by bringing together the elements of a new approach to forensic work, were largely won. A new era dawned in which the near celebrity status of the pathologist gave way to teamwork and the advances they had made were taken to new levels of crime scene investigation, requiring specially equipped laboratories and sophisticated technical resources. Addressing police officers in the preface to his book, *The Investigation of Violence*, he underlined the importance of leaving no stone unturned and concluded, 'We deserve only the reputation we earn'. Keith Simpson certainly earned his reputation and an American colleague, Dr Milton Helpern, Chief Medical Examiner for New York City, said that the informed mind is able to look, observe and react when the bell rings. He added, 'The bell always rings with Keith Simpson'.

GLOSSARY

THE TERMS DEFINED HERE reflect contemporary knowledge and use during the greater part of the twentieth century. Huge advances have been made in forensic pathology in recent years with the emergence of new techniques and procedures. This process of natural development has been aided by the advent of more sophisticated serology and toxicology and, of course, DNA profiling and information management. A new forensic landscape has been created and, with it, a new vocabulary. By accessing expertise in a wide range of new disciplines, such as forensic odontology, entomology and anthropometry, today's forensic practitioners can call on an unprecedented bank of knowledge with its own terminology. In part, this is the legacy of the pioneering forensic pathologists who initiated new realms of discovery and understanding.

ADIPOCERE: Condition of a human corpse when natural body fat solidifies into a yellowish-white, waxy substance. This occurs when a body has been exposed to a damp, airless environment. It is a slow process, also known as saponification, when the neutral body fats are hydrolysed into a mixture of fatty acids and soap. Adipocere adheres to the bones and tends to maintain the shape of the body.

ARSENIC: An irritant poison with a sinister history. White arsenious oxide was at one time used in a variety of products, such as weedkiller, sheep dip and rat poison, regularly employed by gardeners and farmers. The Arsenic Act of 1851 controlled sales and required white arsenic to be mixed with a colourant to distinguish it from commodities such as sugar, salt and flour and thereby prevent accidental poisoning. Purchasers were required to sign the pharmacist's Poisons Register.

Acute arsenical poisoning causes vomiting and diarrhoea, while chronic poisoning involves weight loss, general debility, peripheral neuritis and pigmentation of the skin. A characteristic of arsenic once it enters the body is that it lingers in the hair and fingernails, thereby enabling toxicologists to map the course of poisoning. A minimum lethal dose of arsenic is 2 to 3 grains.

ASPHYXIA: Interference with the respiratory function which restricts breathing and oxygen intake, leading to death. Suffocation, strangulation, choking and drowning are among the causes. Post-mortem indications include cyanosis, congestion of the blood vessels, lividity and petechial haemorrhages in the skin, eyes, and membranes of the heart and lungs.

BLOOD GROUPS: Every human individual's blood falls into one of four internationally recognised groups, designated, A, B, AB and O. These characteristics were defined by Dr Karl Landsteiner in 1900 and are the basis of blood grouping. The individual groups are a function of the red blood cells and the presence in them of agglutinogen. Each group forms a distinct proportion of the population, with AB the most rare at 3 per cent. Every individual's blood group characteristics are inherited and are an unalterable part of that person's identity.

CARBON MONOXIDE POISONING: When breathed in, carbon monoxide combines with haemoglobin in the blood and inhibits its capacity to carry oxygen around the body. Poisoning results once the life-sustaining supply of oxygen is diminished. Death from carbon monoxide poisoning produces a characteristic cherry-red colouring of the skin. This develops as the blood in the underlying vessels changes colour. Blood samples are taken by the pathologist for chemical and spectroscopic tests and, particularly, analysis for the presence of carboxyhaemoglobin (HbCO).

CORONER: The office of coroner is one of the oldest legal appointments in England, dating back to the reign of King Richard I, around 1200. Originally charged with enquiring into any felony, a coroner's duties have, since 1887, been concerned with enquiries into deaths where the circumstances are sudden, violent or unnatural. A coroner must be a solicitor, barrister or medical practitioner and the proceedings he presides over are an inquest or enquiry and not a trial. The law whereby a coroner's court had authority to find a person guilty of murder or manslaughter was abolished in 1977 with the introduction of the Criminal Law Act.

CYANOSIS: Condition in which the skin of the face and extremities of the body take on a bluish tinge due to interference with breathing, blockage of the airways and lack of oxygen entering the lungs. It is a feature of asphyxia.

DUM-DUM BULLETS: Expanding bullets are intended to reduce penetration when they hit their target and massively increase wound damage. They are so named after the Dum-dum arsenal in India where they were first contrived by the British military. Soft-nosed bullets can be modified by cutting a cross-shape in the lead using a knife or saw. Such ammunition was first used at the Battle of Omdurman in 1898 by the British forces under the command of General Kitchener. The Hague Convention in 1899 prohibited the military use of dum-dum ammunition.

EXHUMATION: Disinterring or exhuming a buried body is often a necessary procedure in the course of a murder enquiry. Disputed cause of death or questions about identity may also necessitate exhumation. For an exhumation request to be granted, authorisation is required from a coroner or the Home Office. The procedure may prove significant in cases of suspected poisoning where analysis of organs and tissue samples from the exhumed corpse reveal traces of poisonous substances.

FORENSIC BALLISTICS: The possibility of relating bullets to the weapons that fired them was verified in 1889 by a French scientist, Alexandre Lacassagne. He successfully matched the rifling marks in a bullet taken from a victim's body, with the rifling grooves in the barrel of the murder weapon. From these beginnings, forensic ballistics grew into an exact science, more descriptively known as firearms examination. The investigation of a crime scene shooting includes determining the respective positions of victim and shooter, examining the wounds inflicted and microscopic study of bullets, cartridge cases and propellants. Minute examination of crime weapons, their rifling pattern and other characteristics, adds further forensic detail to aid crime investigation.

FORENSIC MEDICINE: The application of every aspect of medical knowledge to meet legal requirements is called forensic medicine or medical jurisprudence. Forensic comes from the Latin word, *forensis,* meaning 'of the forum' and referring to the principle of making public the cause of death when a person dies. Since its earliest days as a branch of medicine, the field has broadened to include many other scientific disciplines as well as psychiatry, dentistry and anthropology. The job of the forensic pathologist is to determine cause of death and define the supporting medical facts which may be required in the interpretation of evidence in court.

GRAIN: Supposedly named after a grain of wheat and dating back four centuries, this is the smallest unit of mass in the English system. It was incorporated in the apothecaries' weights used by pharmacists in the nineteenth century but is now obsolete, being superceded by the introduction of metric measurements in the 1960s. One grain is equivalent to 65 milligrams.

HISTOLOGY: Microscopic study of the cellular structure of the tissues of the body. Thin sections of tissue are mounted on glass slides and stained with chemicals to highlight their detailed structure and any irregularities. Histological examination of tissue samples taken at post-mortem is a routine pathological procedure.

HYOID BONE: A horseshoe-shaped bone located at the base of the tongue and above the thyroid cartilage in the larynx or voice box. It has four projections or horns, called the greater and lesser cornua. These may break in cases of strangulation when pressure is put on the larynx. A broken hyoid bone is a feature that forensic pathologists look for in cases of suspected strangulation.

HYOSCINE: A vegetable alkaloid belonging to the *Solanaceae* family which includes henbane, belladonna and deadly nightshade. It has been used medicinally to treat anxiety, as its action is to depress the body's central nervous system. Hyoscine is rapidly absorbed through the mucous membranes when a fatal dose causes respiratory failure and stops the heart. A fatal dose may be as low as 8 to 10 milligrams. It is sometimes called scopolamine and referred to as a 'truth drug'.

LIVIDITY: Also known as *Livor mortis*, hypostasis or, simply, as post-mortem staining. It is a process which begins immediately after death when the blood in the body sinks to the lowest point. When the heart stops pumping, blood coagulates in the veins and arteries giving rise to livid patches on the skin. Lividity occurs in the underlying parts of the body which are not in contact with a hard surface, typically the back of the neck, the thighs and small of the back. The internal organs are also affected, as gravity causes the blood to flow down to the lowest parts. The significance of lividity to the forensic examiner is that it helps to determine whether or not a body has been moved after death.

MARSH TEST: In 1836, James Marsh, a scientist working at Woolwich Arsenal, developed a method for identifying arsenic. By converting traces of arsenic into arsine gas and directing it onto a polished surface, he produced a metallic deposit or mirror. The test, which is highly sensitive and capable of detecting very small traces of arsenic, represented a breakthrough in the investigation of cases where poisoning was suspected.

PETECHIAE: Small haemorrhages, also called Tardieu spots, after the French doctor who first described them in 1870. The appearance of petechial haemorrhages in the skin of the face and on the heart and lungs is indicative of death by asphyxia. Severe compression of veins in the neck, or a struggle to breathe, causes the capillaries to burst and form these tiny, but distinctive, effusions of blood.

PHOSPHORUS POISONING: An irritant poison in its yellow form traditionally used in the manufacture of matches and products to kill vermin. By contrast, red phosphorus is inert. Phosphorus poisoning creates symptoms similar to those of a bilious attack; burning sensation in the throat, vomiting and diarrhoea. A feature of such poisoning is the smell of garlic. This is evident in the breath of a person suffering poisonous effects and is also noticeable once the body cavity is opened for post-mortem examination. The pathological appearance of the internal organs may simulate natural disease. Petechiae are observed on the lungs and the liver is enlarged. A fatal does is around 2 grains.

POST-MORTEM: The post-mortem examination, also known as an autopsy or necropsy, is an important procedure carried out by the forensic pathologist to determine cause of death. In 1861, Dr William Guy, Professor of Forensic Medicine at King's College, London, noted what he called 'The great rule to be observed in conducting post-mortems'. It was, 'to examine every cavity and every important organ of the body . . . ', to which he added, 'even when the cause of death is obvious'. His point was that any omission could be exploited later in court to suggest that cause of death lay in some uninvestigated part of the body.

PRECIPITIN TEST: In 1901, Dr Paul Uhlenhuth, a German scientist, developed the first test capable of distinguishing human from animal blood. By injecting protein from chicken eggs into rabbits, which responded by producing anti-bodies, he developed a serum whereby proteins in blood are precipitated and can be identified. A drop of anti-human serum is added to suspect blood which will precipitate if it is of human origin. His achievement represented a breakthrough in the scientific investigation of crime. The test is extremely sensitive and requires only a small sample of blood.

RIGOR MORTIS: After death, the muscles of the body become rigid and fixed in a rigor, hence the term 'stiff' to describe a corpse. This is one of the classic signs of death which arises from coagulation of protein and shortening of the muscles. It is evident first in the eyelids and lower jaw and spreads progressively throughout the body. The process starts within five hours of death and is complete within twelve to eighteen hours. It then slowly disappears as chemical changes occur prompting the onset of decomposition. The state of rigor mortis as an indication of time of death is taken into consideration by the forensic examiner.

STATUS LYMPHATICUS: The thymus gland, located in the upper part of the chest, is a ductless organ chiefly concerned with the body's immune responses. It reaches its full size at the age of two years and then gradually shrinks. Enlargement of the thymus and associated lymph nodes can predispose a child to sudden, unexpected death. Overgrowth of the thymus may put pressure on related parts of the nervous system and blood supply. In association with other factors, such as shock, this condition may result in sudden death. Doctors disagree about the nature of status lymphaticus, but the generally accepted view is that it cannot by itself be a cause of death.

TIME OF DEATH (TOD): This is one of the first questions confronting the forensic pathologist. While lividity and rigor mortis may be taken into account, the most reliable means of establishing TOD is to measure the rate of body cooling. Rectal temperature is measured at timed intervals, using a low-reading thermometer. A rule-of-thumb guide is that a body will lose 1.5 degrees F of heat every hour. The rate of cooling depends on many variable factors; whether the body is clothed, its physical condition (well-nourished or obese), the presence of disease, and environmental factors, such as indoors or out, and season of the year. The examiner plots a graph from timed temperature recordings to establish the rate of cooling and arrive at an estimated TOD.

VITAL REACTION: The pathologist will seek to establish whether injuries on a body were inflicted before, or sustained after, death. When the body receives an injury, its natural defences respond by sending white blood cells (leucocytes) to the site to fight infection and repair damaged tissues. This is known as vital reaction. Microscopic examination of tissue samples taken from the injury site will help to determine whether the wound was caused ante-mortem or post-mortem. Where vital reaction is evident, the injury will have been caused during life.

BIBLIOGRAPHY

BOOKS

Bailey, Guy: *The Fatal Chance*, London (1969)

Barker, Dudley: *Lord Darling's Famous Cases*, London (1936)

Becchofer Roberts, C.E.: *Sir Travers Humphreys: His Career and Cases*, London (1936)

Bedford, Sybille: *The Best We Can Do*, London (1958)

Blundell, R.H. and Wilson, G. Haswell (Eds): *Trial of Buck Ruxton*, Edinburgh (1937)

Bosanquet, Sir Ronald: *The Oxford Circuit*, London (1936)

Bowen, David: *Body of Evidence*, London (2003)

Bresler, Fenton: *Lord Goddard*, London (1977)

Browne, Douglas G. and Tullett, E.V.: *Sir Bernard Spilsbury: His Life and Cases*, London (1951)

Butler, Ivan: *Trials of Donald Hume*, London (1976)

Byrne, Gerald: *John George Haigh: Acid Bath Killer*, London (n.d.)

Camps, Francis E.: with Barber, Richard: *The Investigation of Murder*, London (1966)

Camps, Francis E.: *Medical and Scientific Investigations in the Christie Case*, London (1966)

Camps, Francis E.: *Camps on Crime*, Newton Abbot (1973)

Camps, Francis E. (Ed.): *Gradwohl's Legal Medicine*, Bristol (1976)

Casswell, J.D.: *A Lance for Liberty*, London (1961)

Cherrill, Fred: *Cherrill of The Yard*, London (1954)

Connell, Nicholas: *Walter Dew: The Man Who Caught Crippen*, London (2005)

Cornwell, Rupert: *God's Banker*, London (1983)

Cullen, Tom: *Crippen: The Mild Murderer*, London (1977)

Devlin, Patrick: *Easing the Passing*, London (1985)

Dew, Walter: *I Caught Crippen*, London (1938)

Dewes, Simon: *Doctors of Murder*, London (1962)

Eddowes, John: *The Two Killers of Rillington Place*, London (1954)

Erzinclioglu, Z.: *Forensics*, London (2006)

Evans, Colin: *The Father of Forensics*, London (2007)

Fabian, Robert: *Fabian of The Yard*, London (1950)

Felstead, S.T.: *Sir Richard Muir*, London (1927)

Foot, Paul: *Who Killed Hanratty?*, London (1971)

Furneaux, Rupert: *The Two Stranglers of Rillington Place*, London (1961)

Gaute, J.H.H. and Odell, Robin: *Murder Whatdunit*, London (1982)

Gaute, J.H.H. and Odell, Robin: *Ladykillers 2*, London (1981)

Glaister, John and Brash, James Couper: *Medico-Legal Aspects of the Ruxton Case*, London (1937)

Glaister, John: *The Power of Poison*, London (1954)

Glaister, John: *Final Diagnosis*, London (1964)

Goodman, Jonathan: *The Crippen File*, London (1985)

Graham, Evelyn: *Lord Darling and his Famous Trials*, London (1929)

Grice, Edward: *Great Cases of Sir Henry Curtis Bennett*, London (1937)

Gurney, Larry: *The Calvi Affair*, London (1983)

Haines, Max: *Bothersome Bodies*, Toronto (1988)

Haines, Max: *Canadian Crimes*, Toronto (1998)

Hallworth, Rodney and Williams, Mark: *Where There's a Will...*, London (1983)

Hastings, Macdonald: *The Other Mr Churchill*, London (1963)

Helpern, Milton with Knight, Bernard: *Autopsy*, New York (1977)

Hill, Paull: *Portrait of a Sadist*, London (1960)

Humphreys, Sir Travers: *A Book of Trials*, London (1953)

Humphreys, Christmas: *Both Sides of the Circle*, London (1978)

Hyde, H. Montgomery: *Norman Birkett: The Life of Lord Birkett of Ulverston*, London (1964)

Hyde, H. Montgomery: *Lord Reading (Rufus Isaacs)*, London (1967)

Jackson, Robert: *A Case for the Prosecution: A Biography of Sir Archibald Bodkin*, London (1962)

Jackson, Robert: *Coroner: The Biography of Sir Bentley Purchase*, London (1963)

Jackson, Robert: *The Crime Doctors*, London (1966)

Jackson, Robert: *Francis Camps*, London (1975)

Jackson, Stanley: *The Life and Cases of Mr Justice Humphreys*, London (1955)

Kennedy, Ludovic: *Ten Rillington Place*, London (1961)

La Bern, Arthur: *The Life and Death of a Lady Killer*, London (1967)

La Bern, Arthur: *Haigh: The Mind of a Murderer*, London (1973)

Leach, Charles E: *On Top of the Underworld*, London (1933)

Lebourdais, Isabel: *The Trial of Steven Truscott*, London (1966)

Lefebure, Molly: *Evidence for the Crown*, London (1975)

Lucas, Norman: *The Lucan Mystery*, London (1975)

Lustgarten, Edgar: *The Chalkpit Murder*, London (1974)

Lyons, Frederick J: *George Joseph Smith*, London (1935)

Marham, Patrick: *Trail of Havoc*, London (1987)

Marjoribanks, Edward: *The Life of Sir Edward Marshall Hall*, London (1929)

Montague, Ewan: *The Man Who Never Was*, London (1953)

Moore, Sally: *Lucan:Not Guilty*, London (1987)

Morris, Terence and Blom-Cooper, Louis: *A Calendar of Murder*, London, 1964

Muncie, William: *Crime Pond*, Edinburgh (1979)

Napley, Sir David: *Not Without Prejudice*, London (1982)

Narborough, Fred: *Murder on My Mind*, London (1959)

Neustatter, W. Lindesay: *The Mind of the Murderer*, London (1957)

Oddie, S. Ingleby: *Inquest*, London (1941)

Odell, Robin: *Exhumation of a Murder*, London (1975)

Odell, Robin: *Landmarks in 20th Century Murder*, London (1995)

Oswald, H.R.: *Memoirs of a London County Coroner*, London (1936)

Picton, Bernard: *Murder, Suicide or Accident*, London (1971)

Randall, Leslie: *The Famous Cases of Sir Bernard Spilsbury*, London (1936)

Reading, Marquess: *Rufus Isaacs*, London (1942)

Rentoul, Gervais: *This is My Case*, London (n.d.)

Rentoul, E. and Smith H.: *Glaister's Medical Jurisprudence and Toxicology*, Edinburgh (1973)

Rose, Andrew: *Lethal Witness*, Stroud (2007)

Russell, Lord: *Deadman's Hill:Was Hanratty Guilty?*, London (1965)

Saunders, Kenneth C.: *The Medical Detectives*, London (2001)

Simpson, Keith: *Forensic Medicine*, London (1969)

Simpson, Keith: *Police:The Investigation of Violence*, Plymouth (1978)

Simpson, Keith: *Forty Years of Murder*, London (1978)

Smith, Sir Sydney: *Mostly Murder*, London (1959)

Smith, Sir Sydney and Fiddes, Frederick Smith: *Forensic Medicine*, London (1949)

Taylor, Bernard and Knight, Stephen: *Perfect Murder*, London (1987)

Totterdell, G.H.: *Country Copper*, London (1956)

Tullett, Tom: *Portrait of a Bad Man*, London (1956)

Tullett, Tom: *Strictly Murder*, London (1979)

Whittington-Egan, Richard A.: *The Riddle of Birdhurst Rise*, London (1975)

Willcox, Philip H.: *The Detective Physician*, London (1970)

Williams, John: *Hume: Portrait of a Double Murderer*, London (1960)

Wood, Stuart: *Shades of the Prison House*, London (1932)

Young, Filson (Ed.): *The Trial of Hawley Harvey Crippen*, Edinburgh (1920)

NEWSPAPERS

Blackwood's Magazine
Bombay Medical News Guide
British Medical Journal
Daily Express
Daily Mail
Daily Sketch
Dublin Medical Journal
Glasgow Herald
News of the World
Sunday Telegraph
The Lancet
The Law Journal
The Sunday Times

INDEX OF NAMES

ADAMS, Dr John Bodkin, 153–5, 158

AITCHISON, Lord, 45, 140–2

ALLISON, Dr Andrew, 88, 135

ALNESS, Lord, 88

ALPHON, Peter, 195

ARMSTRONG, Herbert Rowse, 32–5

ARMSTRONG, Janet, 156–7

ARMSTRONG, John, 156–7

ARMSTRONG, Katharine, 32–5

ATTENBOROUGH, Richard, 160

AVARNE, Dr Claude, 89–92

BAILEY, Guy, 196

BANKES, Isabella, 17

BARBER, Richard, 166

BARROW, Eliza, 20–2

BELL, Dr Joseph, 66, 73

BENSON, Gail, 200

BENTLIF, Dr Philip, 90–1

BIRKETT, Sir Norman, 54–5, 85–7, 99, 125–6, 166

BLAMPIED, Dr Philip, 90–1

BODKIN, Sir Archibald, 28, 38

BONATI, Minnie, 46–7

BOSHEARS, Willis Eugene, 163–4

BOURNE, Dr Aleck, 92–3

BOWEN, Professor David, 197, 206

BOYD, Leslie, 207

BRABIN, Mr Justice, 150

BRADY, Patrick, 98

BRASH, Professor James Couper, 99, 119, 128, 143, 173

BRESLER, Fenton, 185

BRITTLE, William, 197–9

BRONTE, Dr Robert, 38–40, 46, 47–8, 49, 50, 59

BROOKS, Dr David, 168

BROWN, Dr Berkeley, 168

BROWN, Dr F. Gordon, 166

BUCHANAN, Mary, 172, 189

BUCKINGHAM, John William, 184

BUCKNILL, Mr Justice, 22, 25

BURNHAM, Alice, 26, 29

CALVI, Carlo, 206

CALVI, Roberto, 203–6

CAMERON, Elsie, 38–9, 41

CAMERON, John QC, 136

CAMERON, Lord, 108

CAMPS, Professor Francis, 10, 41, 42, 102, 103, 107, 109, 143, 172, 182, 185, 191, 198, 199, 207
CARMAN, George QC, 205
CARRAHER, Patrick, 129–130
CASSELS, Sir James Dale KC, 39, 40, 41, 50, 60
CHANTRELLE, Elizabeth, 138–9
CHANTRELLE, Eugene, Marie, 138–9
CHAPMAN, Chief Inspector William, 176, 177, 179
CHERRILL, Chief Superintendent Fred, 147, 178, 179, 180
CHRISTIE, Ethel, 148
CHRISTIE, John Reginald Halliday, 10, 148–150, 179, 182
CHRISTOFI, Hella, 151
CHRISTOFI, Styllou, 151
CHURCHILL, Robert, 44–5, 77, 79
COLERIDGE, Lord, 137
CONSTABLE, Jean, 163–4
COWBURN, Douglas, 55
CRAXI, Bettino, 205
CRIPPEN, Cora, 13–16
CRIPPEN, Dr Hawley Harvey, 13–16, 19
CRUM BROWN, Dr, 139
CURTIS-BENNETT, Sir Henry KC, 33–5, 37, 38, 60
CUSACK, Ralph QC, 198

DARLING, Lord, 33–5
DAVIDSON, Dr James, 97
DAVIES, Dr Gordon, 205
De ANTIQUIS, Alec, 57
DERRY, Professor Douglas, 115
De SARAM, Dr G.W., 199,103–5
DEVLIN, Patrick, 155
DOBKIN, Harry, 128,173
DOBKIN, Rachel, 128

DONALD, Jeannie, 93–5
DOUTHWAITE, Dr Arthur, 154
DOYLE, Sir Arthur Conan, 66, 153, 207
DRENNAN, Professor Murray, 90
DUFF, Edmund Creighton, 47–9
DU PARCQ, Herbert KC, 85–7
DURAND-DEACON, Olive, 189–91

ELMORE, Belle (Mrs Crippen), 13
EMERSON, Ralph Waldo, 143
EMMETT-DUNNE, Frederick, 151, 153, 198
EVANS, Beryl, 148
EVANS, Dr Gerald, 197–8, 162–3
EVANS, Geraldine, 148, 182
EVANS, Timothy John, 149–50, 182

FABIAN, Superintendent Robert, 57
FEARNLEY-WHITTINGSTALL, William, 48
FINLAY, Mr Justice, 39, 40
FOX, Rosaline, 49–50, 60
FOX, Sidney, 49–50, 60, 79–82, 105
FRASER, Dr Thomas, 139
FRENCH, Dr Frank, 27, 29
FYFE, Sir David Maxwell, 125

GALL, Chrissie, 87–9, 163
GARDNER, Dr Eric, 58, 174, 183, 184–5, 186
GARDNER, Margery, 179
GAUTE, Joe, 206, 207
GLAISTER, Professor John, 10, 42, 43, 44, 45, 60, 78, 82, 95, 99, 102, 144, 166, 173, 185
GLYN-JONES, Mr Justice, 164
GODDARD, Lord Chief Justice, 130
GORDON, John, 130
GORRINGE, Margaret, 186

GRADWOHL, Dr Rutherford, 167, 170
GRAVELLE, Philip O., 75
GREENWOOD, Harold, 31
GREGSTON, Michael, 194–5
GUSTAFSON, Dr Gosta, 186

HAIGH, John George, 10, 179, 189–92, 196, 207
HAINES, Max, 169
HALL, Sir Edward Marshall KC, 22, 23, 24, 28, 30, 32, 38, 60
HAMBROOK, Superintendent Walter, 79
HAMILTON, Dr H., 69–70
HAMPSHIRE, Mary, 123–4
HANRATTY, James, 194–5
HARPER, Lynne, 167–9
HARRISON, Professor Richard, 149
HARVEY, Leslie, 107
HARVEY, Sarah, 107–8, 161
HARVEY, Dr Warren, 187–8
HASTINGS, Macdonald, 79
HAY, Gordon, 187–8
HEARN, Sarah Ann, 82–6
HEATH, Neville, George Clevely, 10, 179–80
HEILBRON, Rose QC, 158
HELPERN, Dr Milton, 169, 208
HIGGINS, Patrick, 68–9
HINCKS, Dr Thomas, 33
HOGG, Quintin QC, 198
HOLMES, Reg, 98
HUME, Brian Donald, 147–8, 153
HULLETT, Gertrude, 153–4
HUMPHREYS, Christmas QC, 153
HUMPHREYS, Sir Travers, 15, 22

IRVINE, Dr James, 135
ISAACS, Sir Rufus, 22, 23

JACKSON, Robert, 155, 165
JOWITT, Sir William, 50, 81

KAYE, Emily Beilby, 37
KAYE, Violet, 54–5
KEITH, Lord, 136
KENNEDY, Ludovic, 150
KERR, Dr Douglas, 79
KNIGHT, Frances, 197–108, 162
KNIGHT, Professor Bernard, 169

LANE, Lord, 205
LAW, Andrew Bonar, 35
LAWRENCE, Geoffrey QC, 154
LAWTON, Sir Frederick, 166
LEBOURDAIS, Isabel, 168–9
LEFEBURE, Molly, 172, 173, 175
LE NEVE, Ethel, 14
LEONARD, Oliver James, 157, 159
LEY, Thomas, John, 184, 186
LITTLEJOHN, Professor Harvey, 24, 44, 64, 66, 68, 72, 77, 78, 79, 114, 138
LOCARD, Dr Edmond, 113, 133
LOFTY, Margaret, 26, 29
LUCAS, Dr Arthur, 70
LUCAN, Lady, 201–3
LUCAN, Lord, 201–3
LUFF, Dr Arthur, 15, 17
LYNCH, Dr Gerald Roche, 47, 48, 60, 83, 85, 86

MACKIE, Professor Thomas, 96
MAHON, Patrick, 35, 54–5
MacLAGAN, Dr Douglas, 139
McCLUSKEY, Catherine, 135–7
McINTYRE, Archie, 130, 132
McKENNY-HUGHES, Professor, 96
McMILLAN, Margaret, 139–42
McMILLAN, Robert Brennan, 139–42

McNAGHTEN, Sir Melville, 15
MALIK, Abdul, 199–201
MANCINI, Tony (Lois England), 54–5
MANNINGHAM-BULLER, Sir
    Reginald, 155
MANTON, Bertie, 177–9
MANTON, Caroline, 177–9
MARSHALL, Doreen, 180
MARTIN, Dr Gilbert, 119, 122
MARTIN, Oswald, 34–5
MARYMONT, Marcus, 142, 157,
    159–61
MARYMONT, Mary, 142
MATTHEW, Sir Theobald, 150
MEARNS, Dr Alexander, 125
MEGNIN, Jean-Pierre Dr, 198
MERRETT, Bertha, 43–5, 77, 114
MERRETT, John Donald (Ronald
    Chesney), 43–5, 77
MILLAR, Dr W. Gilbert, 99
MORRELL, Edith, 154–5
MUDIE, John McBain, 183–6
MUIR, Sir Richard, 15
MUNCIE, Chief Superintendent
    William, 187–8
MUNDY, Bessie, 26, 28, 29
MYSZKA, Stanislaw, 131–3

NAPLEY, Sir David, 159, 161, 165, 166,
    170, 204, 205
NARBOROUGH, Chief Inspector
    Fred, 188–91
NEIL, Chief Inspector Arthur Fowler,
    22, 26, 30
NEUSTATTER, Dr W Lindesay, 182
NICKOLLS, Dr Lewis, 149, 157 160

ODDIE, S. Ingleby, 42
O'DWYER, Sir Michael, 56
OSWALD, H.R., 42

PAUL, Dr David, 204, 205
PEACOCK, Linda, 186–8
PENISTAN, Dr John, 167–9
PEPPER, Dr Augustus J., 15, 18, 19
PETTY, Dr Charles, 169
PIERREPOINT, Albert, 38, 133
POLLOCK, Sir Ernest KC, 33
PRIESTLEY, Helen, 92–7
PRIESTLEY, John, 92–7
PURCHASE, Sir Bentley, 13, 42, 57,
    58, 146, 155, 161, 166

QUEEN, Peter, 87–9

RADFORD, Frederick, 191–2
RADFORD, Margery, 191–2
RADZINOWITZ, Professor Leon, 165,
    170
RENTOUL, Sir Gervais KC, 23
RICHARDS, Dr Robert, 93–4
RIVETT, Sandra, 201–3
ROBERTSON, James Ronald, 135–7
ROBINSON, John, 46
ROCHE, Berthe, 31
ROCHE, Mr Justice, 85
ROGERSON, Mary Jane, 118–28
ROUSE, Alfred, Arthur, 51–3
ROWLATT, Mr Justice, 81
RUSSELL, Lord, 130
RUXTON, Dr Buck, 99–100,118–
    28,143,173
RUXTON, Isabella, 99–100
RYFFEL, Dr John, 47

SANGRET, August, 174–5, 196
SAUNDERS, Dr Graham, 82–3
SCHRODER, Sir Walter, 42
SCOTT-DUNN, Jean, 180
SCRUTTON, Mr Justice, 30
SEDDON, Frederick Henry, 19–24

SETTY, Stanley, 147–8

SHAWCROSS, Hartley QC, 125

SHENNAN, Professor Theodore, 93

SHORT, Dr R.D.H., 58

SIMON, Sir Jocelyn, 163

SIMPSON, Professor Keith, 42, 55, 56, 60, 76, 102, 103, 108, 128, 144, 145, 146, 149, 154, 156, 157, 167, 168–70

SINDONA, Michele, 205

SINGH, Udham, 56

SINGLETON, Mr Justice, 125, 179

SKELHORN, Sir Norman, 157

SKERRIT, Joe, 200

SMETHURST, Dr Thomas, 17–18

SMITH, George Joseph, 26–30

SMITH, James, 98–9

SMITH, Lawrence John, 98–9

SMITH, Madeleine, 26–30

SMITH, Sir Sydney, 24, 41, 43, 44, 59, 60, 114, 115, 128, 139–40, 144, 159, 162, 163, 182, 196, 206

SORN, Lord, 132–3

SPILSBURY, Sir Bernard, 64, 78, 79–81, 87, 90, 91–7, 99, 102, 103, 105, 114, 143, 144, 145, 163, 165, 170, 172, 173, 175, 182, 185, 206, 207

SPOONER, Detective Inspector Reginald, 190

STACK, Sir Lee, 41, 62–4, 75

STARCHFIELD, Willie, 25

STILWELL, Thomas, 188

STORIE, Valerie, 194–5

SYDNEY, Vera, 47–9

SYDNEY, Violet, 47–9

TAYLOR, Dr Alfred Swaine, 18–21, 77, 196

TAYLOR, Cynthia, 159, 161

TEARE, Dr Donald, 145, 146, 149, 150, 166, 172, 182, 198, 207

THOMAS, Alice, 82–6

THOMAS, Peter, 197–9

THOMAS, William, 82–3

THORNE, Norman, 38–40, 41

THORWALD, Jurgen, 75,97

TIFFIN, Sydney, 146

TOTTERDELL, Chief Superintendent G.H., 146

TRENCHARD, Lord, 97, 128

THURSTON, Dr Gavin, 202

TRIST, Arthur, 193–4

TRIST, Patricia, 193–4

TRUSCOTT, Steven, 167–9, 199

UHLENHUTH, Dr Paul, 113

VOISIN, Louis, 31

WAITE, Charles E., 75

WAITE, William, 142

WALL, F.C., 132–3

WATTERS, Reginald, 151–2

WEBSTER, Dr John, 49

WHITTINGTON-EGAN, Richard, 49

WILLCOX, Sir William, 15, 16, 18, 19, 21, 22, 23, 25, 28, 29, 32, 33, 42

WILLIAMS, Dr Ray, 207

WILSON, Ernest, 158

WILSON, James, 106

WILSON, Mary, 157–9

WOLFE, Pearl, 174–5

WOMACK, Dr Alan, 151

WOOD, Stuart, 30

WOODHOUSE, Joan, 188–91

YELLOWLEES, Dr Henry, 191

ZAGLOUL, Said Pasha, 62–4, 74, 75

If you enjoyed this book, you may also be interested in ...

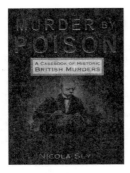

Murder by Poison: A Casebook of Historic British Murders
NICOLA SLY

While there are indeed many infamous female poisoners, such as Mary Ann Cotton, who is believed to have claimed at least twenty victims between 1852 and 1872, men also chose poison as their preferred means to a deadly end. Between 1897 and 1902, George Chapman poisoned three of his lovers with antimony, while William Palmer murdered at least ten victims between 1842 and 1856. Readily obtainable and almost undetectable prior to advances in forensic science during the twentieth century, poisonors rarely stopped at just one victim.

978 0 7524 5065 0

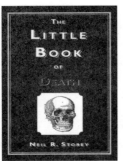

The Little Book of Death
NEIL R. STOREY

This little book is a repository of intriguing, fascinating, obscure, strange and entertaining facts and trivia about the one certainty in all our lives – death. Within this volume are some horrible, unfortunate and downright ludicrous ends. Learn of odd last requests, burials, epitaphs and death rites from around the world, as well as the strange fates of some cadavers – and a whole host of horrible tales about mummies, vampires, zombies and body-snatchers.

978 0 7524 7151 8

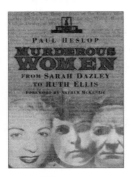

Murderous Women: From Sarah Dazley to Ruth Ellis
PAUL HESLOP

Among the cases featured here are that of Sarah Dazley, hanged in 1843 for poisoning her second husband; Amelia Dyer, the 'baby farmer' who murdered countless numbers of children; Susan Newell, who murdered her newspaper delivery boy; the execution, in 1923, of Edith Thompson for the murder of her husband; and Ruth Ellis, who gunned down her boyfriend outside the Magdala Tavern in 1955, the last woman to lawfully hang in Britain.

978 0 7509 5081 7

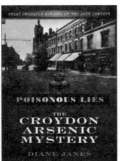

Poisonous Lies: The Croydon Arsenic Mystery
DIANE JANES

In suburban Croydon over a period of ten months during 1928-9, three members of the same family died suddenly. A complex police investigation followed, but no charges were ever brought and the mystery remains officially unsolved. In the eighty years which followed, the finger of suspicion has been pointed at one member of the family after another: now, using the original police files and other contemporary documents, Diane Janes meticulously reconstructs these astonishing events and offers a new solution to an old murder mystery.

978 0 7524 5337 8

Visit our website and discover thousands of other History Press books.

www.thehistorypress.co.uk